Library of Congress Cataloging-in-Publication Data

Fernandez-Botran, Rafael.
Methods in cellular immunology / Rafael Fernandez-Botran, Václav Větvička.—2nd ed.
p. cm.
Includes bibliographical references and index.
ISBN 0-8493-0922-0
1. Cellular immunity—Laboratory manuals. I. Vetvicka, Vaclav. II. Title.
QR185.5 .F47 2001
616.07'9—dc21 2001001524

Direct all inquiries to CRC Press LLC, 2000 N.W. Corporate Blvd., Boca Raton, Florida 33431.

No claim to original U.S. Government works
International Standard Book Number 0-8493-0922-0
Library of Congress Card Number 2001001524
Printed in the United States of America 1 2 3 4 5 6 7 8 9 0
Printed on acid-free paper

Methods in

CELLULAR IMMUNOLOGY

SECOND EDITION

Rafael Fernandez-Botran, Ph.D.
Václav Větvička, Ph.D.

CRC Press
Boca Raton London New York Washington, D.C.

Methods in

CELLULAR IMMUNOLOGY

Dedication

To Anna, Christina, Antonio, and Jana

Preface

The extraordinary advancement of immunology in the past few years has made some techniques obsolete, whereas others have gained widespread use. A variety of novel molecules — including cytokines, chemokines, and surface proteins — have been cloned and characterized while new information has been obtained about the functions and importance of some previously known molecules. In this 2nd edition, changes have been made accordingly, deleting several techniques no longer in use, updating others, and adding new and relevant information and methodology pertaining, especially, to novel cytokines and chemokines. Still, the basic format of the original version has been maintained and the goal remains the same: to make it a useful and easy-to-use tool for investigators employing cellular immunological techniques in their research, regardless of whether or not immunology is their main area of expertise.

Those familiar with the original version will find the same step-by-step coverage of background information, alternative techniques, potential limitations or pitfalls, and other useful information. To make the techniques easier to follow, information regarding manufacturers and commercial sources of chemicals and reagents is also included, as is a comprehensive list of references, thus allowing the reader to refer to the original information and/or techniques. Throughout this book, we have tried to provide techniques for both human and murine models.

Chapter 1 deals with the isolation and preparation of different populations of cells from both human and murine origin. Chapter 2 is dedicated to flow cytometry, including techniques for labeling of antibodies and fluorescent analyses of intracellular Ca^{2+} and cell cycles, as well as new techniques for intracellular staining. In Chapter 3, we cover the preparation and culture of clones of murine and human T cells and human B cells, expanded to include a section on T-cell hybridomas. Chapter 4 deals with the assessment of proliferation by both isotopic and non-isotopic techniques, and Chapter 5 covers cytotoxic cell populations, including assessment of cytotoxic activity, isolation of NK cells, and generation of LAK cells. Chapters 6 and 8, covering cytokines and their receptors, have been updated with new information on novel cytokines. An entirely new section of the assay of chemokines has been incorporated (Chapter 7). Chapters 9 and 10 focus on antibodies — from the generation of polyclonal and monoclonal antibodies, the conjugation of peptides or proteins to carriers, and the detection of antibodies and antibody-producing cells (including ELISA techniques), to the purification and modification of antibodies. The final two chapters cover the preparation of buffers and media, and provide a list of manufacturers, complete with addresses, telephone numbers, and Web pages.

The Authors

Rafael Fernandez-Botran, Ph.D., is an associate professor in the Department of Pathology and Laboratory Medicine, Division of Experimental Immunology and Immunopathology, School of Medicine, University of Louisville, Kentucky. Dr. Fernandez-Botran received his bachelor of science degree in biological chemistry from San Carlos University, Guatemala in 1979 and his Ph.D. in microbiology from the University of Kansas Medical Center, Kansas City in 1985. Dr. Fernandez-Botran worked as a postdoctoral fellow and instructor in the laboratories of Dr. Ellen S. Vitetta and Dr. Jonathan W. Uhr at the Department of Microbiology, University of Texas Southwestern Medical Center, Dallas, where his work centered on the study of cytokines, particularly interleukin-4, and their roles in the proliferation and differentiation of $CD4^{+}$ T cell subsets and B cells, and on the characterization of interleukin-4 receptors and their interactions with interleukin-2 receptors.

More recently, Dr. Fernandez-Botran's major research interests have focused on the immunoregulatory roles of soluble cytokine receptors and the interactions between cytokines and glycosaminoglycans. Dr. Fernandez-Botran has received several fellowships and awards, including the New Investigator Recognition Award from the Clinical Immunology Society (CIS) in 1989, and the President's Young Investigator Award from the University of Louisville in 1993. His research activities have resulted in more than 50 published works, including articles, several reviews, and chapters.

Václav Větvička, Ph.D., is an assistant professor in the Department of Pathology, Division of Experimental Immunology and Immunopathology, School of Medicine, University of Louisville, Kentucky. Dr. Větvička graduated in 1978 from Charles University in Prague, Czech Republic with an advanced degree in biology. He obtained his Ph.D. in 1983 from the Czechoslovak Academy of Sciences, Institute of Microbiology, Prague. He is a member of the Czech Immunological Society, American Association of Immunologists, International Society of Developmental and Comparative Immunology, and American Association for Cancer Research. In 1984 he was awarded the Distinguished Young Scientist Award of the Czechoslovak Academy of Sciences. During 1984 to 1985 and 1988 he spent a total of 18 months as a research associate at the Oklahoma Medical Research Foundation, Oklahoma City.

Dr. Větvička is the author or co-author of more than 160 original papers and several review articles. He is co-author of the books *Evolution of Immune Reactions, Immunology of Annelids, Aspartic Proteinases, Methods in Cellular Immunology, Advanced Methods in Cellular Immunology,* and *Evolutionary Mechanisms of Defense Reactions*, and co-editor of the books *Immunological Disorders in Mice and Immune System Accessory Cells.* Dr. Větvička's current major research interests include the role of procathepsin D in cancer development, the role of glucan in NK cell activation, and the phylogenic aspects of defense reactions. He holds three patents.

Contents

Contents

chapter one

Cells

Contents

I. Preparation of cell suspensions

A. Heat inactivation of fetal calf serum

Materials and reagents

- Fetal calf serum (FCS)
- Thermometer
- Equivalent bottle
- Water bath

Protocol

1. Remove serum from –20°C freezer and allow to thaw overnight in a refrigerator.
2. Fill an equivalent bottle with water and place a thermometer in the water. Fill a water bath to 0.25 in. above the serum line.
3. Preheat the water bath to 56°C. Place the bottles with FCS and a bottle with a thermometer in the water bath.
4. Mix the serum every 10 minutes (min) to avoid gelling of proteins.
5. When the temperature reaches 56°C, begin timing. Heat inactivate for 30 min with mixing continued every 10 min.
6. Cool rapidly by placing on ice.
7. Freeze the entire bottle or smaller aliquots.

Comments

1. The occasional appearance of turbidity or flocculent material does not affect the quality of serum.

B. *Spleen*

Materials and reagents

- RPMI 1640 medium or PBS
- Squeeze bottle with 70% ethanol
- Scissors and forceps
- Cutting board or paper towels
- 60 × 15-mm Petri dishes
- Stainless steel screen (Thomas)
- Glass tissue homogenizer (Fisher)
- Fetal calf serum (FCS)
- 15-ml conical centrifuge tube

Protocol

1. Kill mouse either by cervical dislocation or CO_2 inhalation. Place the mouse on cutting board (or on paper towel) and soak it with ethanol to reduce the possibility of hair becoming airborne.
2. Make a cut through the skin in the inguinal region. With fingers on both sides of the cut, pull toward the tail and head until the peritoneal wall is sufficiently exposed. Soak the peritoneal wall with ethanol.
3. Cut the peritoneal wall, lift the spleen with the forceps, and separate it from connecting tissues with scissors. Put the spleen into a Petri dish containing medium.
4. Cut the spleen into several smaller pieces and make a suspension.
5. Gently tease pieces of tissues over stainless steel screens using the plunger of a 5-ml syringe, or alternatively use a glass homogenizer.
6. Remove large debris and cell clumps by layering the cell suspension over 3 ml heat-inactivated FCS for 10 min on ice. Wash the suspension by centrifugation at 300 × *g* for 10 min at 4°C and keep in medium with at least 5% FCS.

Comments

1. For tissue culture studies, perform the entire isolation in a sterile hood and use only sterile instruments, media, and dishes. Do not cut the peritoneal wall with the same scissors used for cutting the skin.
2. Keep cells on ice.

3. The same procedure can be used for lymph nodes or thymus.
4. Typical yield per normal spleen of an untreated mouse is 5×10^7 to 2.5×10^8 cells, depending on the strain used.

C. *Bone marrow*

Materials and reagents

- RPMI 1640 medium or PBS
- Squeeze bottle with 70% ethanol
- Scissors and forceps
- Cutting board or paper towels
- 60 × 15-mm Petri dishes
- 3-ml syringes
- 22G1 needles
- 15-ml conical centrifuge tube

Protocol

1. Kill mouse either by cervical dislocation or CO_2 inhalation. Place the mouse on its back on cutting board (or on paper towel) and soak it with ethanol to reduce the possibility of hair becoming airborne.
2. Make a long transverse cut through the skin in the middle of the abdominal area. Reflect skin from the hindquarters and the hind legs.
3. Separate the legs from the body at the hip joint; remove the feet. Place the legs in a Petri dish containing medium.
4. Remove all muscle tissue from the femur and tibia, separate femur and tibia, and cut off the epiphyses on both ends.
5. Puncture the bone end with a needle and flush out the bone marrow with 3 ml media.
6. Remove the large debris and cell clumps by layering the cell suspension over 3 ml heat-inactivated FCS for 10 min on ice. Wash the suspension by centrifugation at 300*g* for 10 min at 4°C and keep in medium with at least 5% FCS.

Comments

1. For tissue culture studies, perform the entire isolation in a sterile hood and use only sterile instruments, media, and dishes. Do not use the same scissors used for cutting the skin for muscle removal.
2. Keep cells on ice.
3. Typical yield of cells is 3 to 7×10^7 per mouse.

D. Peritoneal cells

Materials and reagents

- RPMI 1640 medium or PBS
- Squeeze bottle with 70% ethanol
- Scissors and forceps
- Cutting board or paper towels
- 5-ml syringes
- 22G1 and 23G1 needles
- Thioglycollate medium (Fluid Thioglycollate Medium; Becton Dickinson)
- 15-ml conical centrifuge tubes

Protocol

1. Kill mouse either by cervical dislocation or CO_2 inhalation. Place the mouse on its back on cutting board (or on paper towel) and soak it with ethanol to reduce the possibility of hair becoming airborne.
2. Make a cut through the skin in the inguinal region. With fingers on both sides of the cut, pull toward the tail and head until the peritoneal wall is sufficiently exposed. Soak the peritoneal wall with ethanol.
3. Inject 5 ml medium into the peritoneal cavity using a 22G1 needle. Gently massage the peritoneum and slowly draw the fluid using a 23G1 needle. One may need to puncture the cavity in several places. Wash the suspension by centrifugation at 300*g* for 10 min at 4°C and keep in medium with at least 5% FCS.

Comments

1. The average yield is 2×10^6 cells per mouse. Approximately 30 to 40% of cells are macrophages.
2. One can substantially increase the yield of cells (percentage of macrophages will be more than 90%) by injecting 3 ml thioglycollate medium i.p. 3 to 6 days prior to harvesting peritoneal cells. The yield depends on the strain, being between 1×10^7 per mouse (A/J or BALB/c) and 2 to 3×10^7 (C57BL/6, C57BL/10).[1]
3. If using thioglycollate medium, remember three important things:
   a. The macrophages are activated and thus you cannot compare them with macrophages from untreated mice.[1,2]
   b. Always use the same interval between thioglycollate injection and cell harvesting.
   c. Thioglycollate medium is a bacteriological medium; therefore, it must be kept sterile.

E. *Blood collection*

Materials and reagents

- Sterile PBS
- Gauze
- Microhematocrit tubes (Fisher)
- Anesthesia
- Eppendorf tubes
- Anticoagulation agent

Protocol

1. Anesthetize the animal according to the instructions from the Animal Care Facility.
2. Dip the microhematocrit tube into the anticoagulation agent.
3. Introduce the tip of the microhematocrit tube at the medial canthus of the orbital sinus.
4. With axial rotation, slowly and gently advance the tip toward the rear of the socket until the blood starts to flow into the tube.
5. Remove the microhematocrit tube from the orbit and wash excess blood from the site with a gauze moistened in PBS.
6. Transfer the blood into the Eppendorf tube with the anticoagulation agent.

Comments

1. This technique is suitable for small laboratory animals such as mice, rats, or hamsters.

F. *Cell counting*

Materials and reagents

- Cell suspension
- Hemocytometer (Fisher)
- Pipettes
- Pasteur pipettes
- Eppendorf tubes
- Türk or Trypan blue solution

Protocol

1. Dilute cells in either Türk or Trypan blue solution, mix thoroughly, and add one drop into hemocytometer chamber using a Pasteur pipette. Do not overfill or underfill the chamber.

2. Count the cells in the 1-mm center square. Count cells touching the top and left middle lines of the perimeter of each square.
3. Cell counts/ml = Actual number of cells × Dilution factor × 10^4.

Comments

1. It is possible to increase the accuracy by counting more than one 1-mm square (5 to 10 squares). In that case, substitute *Actual number of cells* with *Average number of cells per square.*
2. The optimal cell dilution is approximately 20 to 50 cells per square.

G. *Cell counting using Türk solution*

Materials and reagents

- Cell suspension
- Türk solution
- Hemocytometer
- Pipettes
- Eppendorf tubes

Protocol

1. Dilute cells in Türk solution, mix thoroughly, add one drop into hemocytometer chamber using a Pasteur pipette, and count them.

Comments

1. Türk solution lyses all erythrocytes; thus, it is necessary to use it for counting of either spleen cells or cell suspension resulting from isolation from peripheral blood.

H. *Determination of cell viability*

1. Trypan blue exclusion

Materials and reagents

- Cell suspension at 2 to 6 × 10^6 cells/ml
- Trypan blue (Sigma), 0.4% (w/v) in water
- PBS
- 5-ml glass or plastic tube

Protocol

1. Mix 0.25 ml Trypan blue solution, 0.15 ml PBS, and 0.1 ml cell suspension. Allow to stand for 5 to 15 min.

2. Transfer a small amount of the suspension either to the hemocytometer chamber or on cover glass and count the cells. Nonviable cells will stain blue.

$$\text{Cell viability (\%)} = \frac{\text{Number of viable cells}}{\text{Number of viable cells} + \text{Number of dead cells}} \times 100$$

Comments

1. Trypan blue has a greater affinity for serum proteins than for cellular proteins. If the background is too dark, resuspend the cells in PBS prior to counting.
2. Do not incubate cells in Trypan blue solution longer than 15 min, as viable cells might begin to take up dye.

2. Fluorescein diacetate

Materials and reagents

- Cell suspension at approximately 2×10^6 cells/ml
- Fluorescein diacetate (Sigma), 5 mg/ml in acetone, stored at –20°C
- PBS
- FCS
- Fluorescence microscope or flow cytometer
- 15-ml conical centrifuge tube

Protocol

1. Dilute fluorescein diacetate in PBS at room temperature (1:50). Add 0.1 ml diluted fluorescein diacetate to 0.9 ml cell suspension.
2. Incubate for 5 to 10 min at room temperature. Examine cells with a fluorescence microscope or with a flow cytometer. Viable cells will appear bright green; dead cells will not be stained at all. Determine the percent of viable cells as described above.

Comments

1. Fluorescein diacetate is taken in by all cells but only shows green fluorescence after hydrolyzation inside living cells.
2. This technique is particularly useful in combination with rhodamine- (TRITC) or phycoerythrin-labeled antibodies.

3. Propidium iodide

Materials and reagents

- Cell suspension
- Propidium iodide (Sigma), 1 mg/ml in PBS
- 5-ml centrifuge tubes or 1.5-ml Eppendorf tubes
- Fluorescence microscope or flow cytometer

Protocol

1. Mix 200 µl cells with 10 µl propidium iodide and incubate for 5 min at 4°C.
2. Fill the tube with washing medium and wash twice by spinning 10 min at 200*g*.
3. Examine cells with a fluorescence microscope or with a flow cytometer. Dead cells will appear red; viable cells will not be stained at all. Determine the percent of viable cells as described above.

Comments

1. This technique can be used in combination with fluorescein diacetate.
2. Use propidium iodide staining at time of last incubation in every cell-surface staining experiment using FITC-labeled antibodies and flow cytometer.
3. Do not use in combination with TRITC- or phycoerythrin-labeled antibodies.

I. Removal of erythrocytes from cell suspensions

1. ACK lysing buffer

Materials and reagents

- Cell suspension
- ACK lysing buffer
- 15-ml conical centrifuge tubes

Protocol

1. Add spleen cell suspension into the lysing buffer. Use approximately 5 ml per spleen.
2. Incubate for 5 min at room temperature with occasional gentle shaking.

3. Fill the tube with washing medium (optimally with the medium you plan to use in subsequent experiment), wash 2× by centrifugation for 10 min at 200 × *g*.

2. Hemolytic Gey's solution

Materials and reagents

- Cell suspension
- Gey's solution
- FCS
- 15-ml conical centrifuge tubes

Protocol

1. Add 5 ml Gey's solution to 1 × 10^8 spleen cells and incubate for 5 min on ice.
2. Underlay the cells with 100% FCS and spin at 300 × *g* for 10 min at room temperature. Wash 2× with washing medium by spinning at 300*g* for 10 min at room temperature.

3. Tris-buffered ammonium chloride

Materials and reagents

- Cell suspension
- FCS
- Tris-buffered ammonium chloride
- 15-ml conical centrifuge tube

Protocol

1. Resuspend 1 × 10^8 cells in 3 ml Tris-buffered ammonium chloride (working solution) and incubate for 2 min at room temperature.
2. Underlay the cells with 100% FCS and spin at 300 × *g* for 10 min. Wash 2× with washing medium.

Comments

1. Regardless of which method is used, if the cell suspension still looks red, it is necessary to repeat the entire process.
2. The removal of red blood cells is necessary for spleen cell suspension only.
3. Remove red blood cells before counting the cells.

4. Distilled water

Materials and reagents

- Cell suspension
- 50-ml centrifuge tubes
- Distilled water
- Medium with FCS
- Vortex

Protocol

1. Resuspend 5×10^7 cells in 0.2 ml medium and add 1 ml distilled water.
2. Wait 15 seconds(s) and immediately add 45 ml medium, vortex, and centrifuge at 300*g* for 10 min. Repeat Steps 1 and 2 once or twice according to the level of red cell contamination.

Comments

1. The use of distilled water is by far the easiest technique for red cell removal. The only trick is not to let the cell suspension remain too long in water.

J. Removal of dead cells

1. Centrifugation through FCS

Materials and reagents

- Cell suspension
- FCS
- 15-ml conical centrifuge tube

Protocol

1. Carefully layer 1×10^8 cells in 1 ml medium over 3 ml FCS in a 15-ml conical centrifuge tube. Centrifuge at 300*g* for 10 min.
2. Discard the supernatant and wash the cells twice in an appropriate medium.

2. Centrifugation through Ficoll-Hypaque™

Materials and reagents

- Cell suspension

- Ficoll-Hypaque solution κ = 1.09 (Sigma; Hypaque-76 from Winthrop Pharmaceuticals)
- RMPI 1640 medium with 5% FCS
- 15-ml conical centrifuge tube

Protocol[3]

1. Add 4 ml Ficoll-Hypaque solution to the 15-ml conical tube and carefully layer 4 ml cells (5×10^6 to 1×10^7/ml) over Ficoll-Hypaque (use the wall of the tube).
2. Spin at 2000*g* for 20 min at room temperature with brake off.
3. Collect all the fluid, add medium with FCS, and centrifuge at 300*g* for 15 min at 4°C. Wash 2× in an appropriate medium at 250*g* for 10 min.

Comments

1. The density of the Ficoll-Hypaque mixture is temperature-dependent. It is necessary to use the prewarmed Ficoll-Hypaque (20°C) and centrifuge.

II. Isolation of cells

The ability to fractionate heterologous cell populations according to their cell surface markers or biological or physical properties is essential for a detailed characterization of the properties and characteristics of the particular cell types. Negative selection (i.e., the elimination of a specific cell subset), is a well-established immunological method. Thus, for more than two decades, cells labeled with a specific antibody have been removed from the whole population by the lytic action of the complement.[11] In addition, other techniques based on principles of cell destruction are also used.[12] However, these techniques have an inherent disadvantage. Although specific cell types can be easily removed, the survivors are an enriched but never pure population. Additionaly, the biological functions of survivors are often affected by biologically active substances released from the destroyed cells.[13] Positive selection — unlike its negative counterpart — refers to the direct selection and recovery of cells that express the particular surface marker among a heterogeneous group of cells. Rather than eliminating the undesired cells and leaving the residual population, positive selection means an enrichment, or even purification, of the desired cells. Nevertheless, both the ability of the system to identify the desired cell subpopulation and the mechanics of their subsequent removal from the mixed-cell population must be considered.

A. Isolation of B cells

1. B-cell enrichment by cytotoxic elimination of T cells

Materials and reagents

- Cell suspension
- Antibodies of known specificity and cytotoxic titer
- RPMI 1640 medium with 10% FCS
- Rabbit complement
- 15-ml conical centrifuge tubes

Protocol

1. Dilute cell suspension to 10^7 cells/ml. Add 1 ml antibodies and incubate for 30 min.
2. Wash the cell suspension in medium at 250*g* for 10 min at room temperature.
3. Add 1 ml diluted rabbit complement and incubate for 30 min at 37°C.
4. Wash the cell suspension 3× in medium at 250*g* for 10 min at room temperature.

Comments

1. The optimal antibodies are anti-Thy-1 (in the case of mouse cells) or anti-CD3 (in the case of human cells). The use of either anti-CD4 or anti-CD8 antibodies will result in selective elimination of either $CD4^+$ or $CD8^+$ T cells.[4]

2. Panning[5]

Materials and reagents

- Cell suspension
- Anti-Ig antibody (or anti-CD19, anti-CD20), affinity purified
- PBS
- 15 × 100-mm Petri dishes
- RPMI 1640 medium with 5% FCS

Protocol

1. Coat the Petri dish with 10 ml antibody diluted to 50 to 100 mg/ml. Be sure that the entire surface of the dish is covered. Incubate for 2 hours (hr) at room temperature, or overnight at 4°C.
2. Remove the anti-Ig solution and wash the plate 4× with cold PBS.

3. Add cells (up to 2×10^8) in 5 ml medium with FCS and incubate for 30 min at room temperature.
4. Remove nonadherent cells (T cells).
5. Pour 10 ml medium with FCS.
6. With a pipette or syringe, draw most of the medium off and strongly pour the medium back into one area of the dish. Repeat several times over a new area until the entire dish is covered and most of the cells are removed.

Comments

1. The coated plates can be stored in the refrigerator for up to 4 weeks.
2. The anti-Ig solution can be stored and used repeatedly.
3. This method can also be used for isolation of T cells.
4. Check the efficiency of isolation by staining the final suspension with anti-Ig (anti-CD19/20) or anti-CD3 antibodies conjugated to a fluorescent marker.

3. Isolation of B cells using Percoll gradient

Materials and reagents

- Hanks' balanced salt solution (HBSS)
- Percoll (Pharmacia LKB; Sigma)
- 50-ml polypropylene conical centrifuge tubes
- 15-ml glass centrifuge tubes
- Cell suspension

Protocol

1. Prepare 70% Percoll by mixing 170 ml HBSS with 290 ml Percoll.
2. Prepare 50%, 60%, and 66% Percoll as follows:

	50%	60%	66%
HBSS (ml)	8.58	4.26	1.71
70% Percoll (ml)	21.42	25.74	28.29

3. Prepare a 50%-60%-66%-70% Percoll gradient in 15-ml tubes. Start with 2.5 ml of 70% Percoll; gently overlay 2.5 ml of 66% Percoll, followed by 2.5 ml of 60% Percoll, and finally 2.5 ml of 50% Percoll. Incubate the gradients for 15 min on ice.
4. Gently add 2.5 ml cell suspension (approximately 5×10^7/ml) on top of the gradient.
5. Centrifuge gradients for 13 min at 1900*g* at 4°C.

6. Aspirate HBSS and 50% Percoll and separately collect cells at interfaces between remaining layers.
7. Wash cells 3× with HBSS by centrifugation at 300*g* at 4°C.

Comments

1. Best results are achieved when this method is used as a supplement to any of the previously described methods for enrichment of B-cell populations.
2. Keep HBSS and all Percoll solutions on ice at all times; the success of the separation depends on the temperature.
3. Cells at the 60%-66% Percoll interface are resting B lymphocytes; cells at the 50%–60% Percoll interface are activated B cells.
4. If a sterile cell suspension is needed, perform all steps in a laminar flow hood.

B. *Isolation of T cells*

1. *Adherence to nylon wool*[6]

Materials and reagents

- Cell suspension
- RPMI 1640 medium with 5% FCS
- 50-ml conical centrifuge tubes
- Nylon wool (Polysciences)
- 10-, 30-, or 60-ml disposable syringes
- Three-way stopcock
- HCl (1%)
- Glass beaker

Protocol

1. Boil the nylon wool in 1% HCl in a glass beaker for 20 min. Wait until the fluid is cold and then pour it off. Wash the nylon wool repeatedly to remove all HCl and check the pH. Let the nylon wool dry at room temperature and then weigh in appropriate aliquots. One can store the dry nylon wool indefinitely.
2. Prepare the nylon wool column by packing a syringe of an appropriate size with preboiled nylon wool; 2 g of nylon wool is suitable for separation of approximately 3×10^8 cells in 4 ml.
3. Equilibrate the column by running 10× the loading volume of warm (37°C) medium. Remove all trapped air bubbles by tapping on the column sides. Compact the nylon wool with a pipette.
4. Close the three-way stopcock and add an extra 2 to 3 ml warm medium. Incubate the column for 30 min at 37°C.

5. Drain the column completely and add the prewarmed cell suspension (approximately 7.5 × 10^7 cell/ml).
6. Drain the column, add 1 to 2 ml warm medium, and drain again. Add 3 ml medium to prevent drying and close the stopcock.
7. Incubate the column for another 30 min at 37°C.
8. Fill the column with warm medium, open the stopcock, and collect the first 15 to 20 ml nonadherent cells.
9. Wash the cell suspension 2× in an appropriate medium at 250*g* for 10 min at 4°C.

Comments

1. If a sterile cell suspension is required, perform all steps in a laminar flow hood.
2. Do not overload the column.
3. For further use of nylon wool, repeat Step 1.

2. T-cell enrichment by cytotoxic elimination

Materials and reagents

- Cell suspension
- Antibodies of known specificity and cytotoxic titer
- RPMI 1640 medium with 5% FCS
- Rabbit complement
- 15-ml conical centrifuge tubes

Protocol

1. Dilute cell suspension to 10^7 cells/ml. Add 1 ml antibodies and incubate for 30 min.
2. Wash the cell suspension in medium at 250*g* for 10 min at 4°C.
3. Add 1 ml diluted rabbit complement and incubate for 30 min at 37°C.
4. Wash the cell suspension 3× in medium at 250*g* for 10 min at 4°C.

Comments

1. Several pilot experiments are crucial prior to the actual separation. The optimal conditions vary according to the antibody, cells, and complement used. After establishing the optimal conditions, controls (addition of antibodies without complement and addition of complement without antibodies) need not be routinely performed.
2. The antibodies used depend on the type of cells being eliminated. Anti-MHC class II antibodies and/or anti-CD19 or anti-CD20 antibodies work well for elimination of B cells, anti-CD14 antibodies for elimination of monocytes, and anti-F4/80 antibodies for elimination

of mouse macrophages. The use of purified IgG is not necessary; culture supernatants or ascites fluids work just fine. The optimal concentration must be determined in pilot experiments. The temperature for incubation also varies according to the antibodies used and thus must be determined in pilot experiments.
3. Test the new lot of rabbit complement for spontaneous cytotoxicity (without addition of antibodies). If possible, prepare your own complement (by bleeding the rabbit, incubate serum for 20 min at room temperature, followed by 120 min at 4°C). If you decide to use commercial rabbit complement, the best results are achieved with complement from Cedarlane. After determining the ideal dilution, store aliquots of complement at –80°C for no longer than 1 year. Dilute the complement just before use and always discard the unused part.
4. The temperature for incubation of cells with antibodies also varies according to the antibody used. The authors would recommend performing the first test at 4°C and moving to either room temperature, or even 37°C, but only if the results are not satisfactory.

C. *Isolation of monocytes/macrophages*

1. Adherence to Sephadex G-10[7]

Materials and reagents

- Cell suspension
- RPMI 1640 medium with 5% FCS
- Sephadex G-10 (Pharmacia, Sigma)
- 10- or 50-ml disposable syringe
- Three-way stopcock
- 50-ml conical centrifuge tube
- Nylon wool (Polysciences)
- 1% SDS in PBS
- Pasteur pipette

Protocol

1. Prepare an empty syringe with a closed three-way stopcock and a needle and prewarm the RPMI 1640 medium.
2. Put approximately 10 mg nylon wool into the bottom of the syringe and press well with the tip of a pipette. Add 5 to 10 ml medium with FCS and remove all air bubbles. With the tip of a pipette, or Pasteur pipette, hold the nylon wool firmly down and open the stopcock to seal the syringe. Close the stopcock.
3. Mix Sephadex G-10 with warm (37°C) medium with FCS.
4. Add 5 to 10 ml Sephadex G-10 into the syringe and allow to settle down. Open the stopcock, but do not allow all medium to drain from

the Sephadex G-10 mixture. Add the remainder of the Sephadex G-10 (leave space for approximately 3 ml of cells). Wash the column with 50 to 150 ml warm medium with FCS. Close the stopcock.

5. Add the cell suspension (1×10^8) dropwise onto the column. Open the stopcock and allow the cells to penetrate the column. Close the stopcock and incubate for 30 min at 37°C.
6. Open the stopcock and collect the nonadherent cells. Add additional warm medium, but collect only about 10 to 20 ml (depending on the size of the column).
7. Let the possible contaminating Sephadex G-10 settle in a tube (1 to 2 min), decant the medium into a new tube, and wash the cell suspension in medium at $250 \times g$ for 10 min at 4°C.

Comments

1. If a sterile cell suspension is required, perform all steps in a laminar flow hood.
2. To completely deplete the monocytes/macrophages, repeat the entire process one more time.
3. Collect the used Sephadex G-10. Wash repeatedly with an excess of water. Pour off the water, add a 1% solution of sodium dodecyl sulfate in PBS, and incubate at room temperature for at least 12 hr. Pour off the SDS solution and wash repeatedly with an excess of water (at least 10×). Wash 5× with PBS. Resuspend Sephadex G-10 in a small volume of PBS and store at 4°C. Sephadex G-10 can be used up to five times.

2. Isolation of monocytes by adhesion and cultivation

Materials and reagents

- Peripheral blood
- 3.8% sodium citrate
- 24-well tissue culture plates
- 15-ml and 50-ml conical centrifuge tubes
- Ficoll-Histopaque (Sigma)
- 1 *M* $CaCl_2$
- 6% Dextran T-500 (Sigma)
- Saline
- 16 × 125-mm centrifuge tubes
- Hanks' buffered saline
- RMPI 1640 medium
- Antibiotics
- Trypsin-EDTA solution (BioWhittaker; Intergen)

Protocol

1. Centrifuge freshly drawn peripheral blood with 0.11 ml of 3.8% sodium citrate/ml of blood at 1000*g* at room temperature for 20 min.
2. Remove plasma from cells. Place approximately 8 ml plasma into new tube and spin for 15 min at 1000*g* at room temperature.
3. Add 5 ml of 6% dextran to cells. Bring volume up to 50 ml with saline. Invert several times, loosen cap, and let sit for 30 min at room temperature.
4. Put the remaining plasma into a sterile bottle and add 20 µl $CaCl_2$/ml of plasma (this is now considered to be an autologous serum). Incubate at 37°C for 1 hr.
5. Dilute part of the serum 3× with saline.
6. Remove supernatant from the dextran sedimentation tube and spin at 350*g* for 10 min at room temperature. Discard supernatant and save cells.
7. Resuspend these cells in diluted serum (1 to 4 × 10^6/ml). Place 8 ml cell solution into each of 16 × 125-mm tubes and underlay with 3 ml Ficoll-Histopaque. Centrifuge at 1000*g* for 25 min at room temperature.
8. Monocytes are in the band at the interface of the gradient. Remove this layer, put the cells into a 50-ml tube and fill with cold Hanks' buffered saline. Wash twice by centrifugation at 350*g* for 10 min at 4°C.
9. Dilute cells to 2 to 3 × 10^6/ml with Hanks' buffered saline. Add 0.1% autologous serum (from Step 4) and place 1 ml cells/well in a 24-well tissue culture plate. Incubate for 2 hr at 37°C.
10. Aspirate nonadherent cells, wash once with RPMI 1640, add 2 ml RPMI 1640 medium supplemented with 5% autologous serum and antibiotics, and incubate for 3 to 4 days in a humidified 37°C, 5% CO_2 incubator.
11. Resulting monocytes/macrophages can be removed by Trypsin-EDTA solution (aspirate medium from wells, add 0.2 ml Trypsin-EDTA solution into each well, and incubate for 5 to 10 min at 37°C). Check under the microscope. Pool cells from all wells into a 50-ml tube, add RMPI 1640 medium, and centrifuge at 350*g* for 10 min at 4°C).

Comments

1. The resulting population depends on the time of incubation. It is either a mixture of monocytes and macrophages (with a minor contamination of other cell types) or, in the case of 4-day or longer incubations, it consists of macrophages only.
2. If a sterile cell suspension is required, perform all steps in a laminar flow hood.

3. Isolation of monocytes by adherence

Materials and reagents

- Peripheral blood mononuclear cells
- RMPI 1640 medium
- 75-cm² tissue culture flasks (Corning; Costar)
- 15-ml conical centrifuge tube
- Trypsin-EDTA (BioWhittaker; Intergen) or rubber policeman (Costar)

Protocol

1. Dilute cells in RMPI 1640 medium to a concentration 2×10^6/ml.
2. Put 10 ml diluted cells into 75-cm² tissue culture flask and incubate 60 min in a humidified 37°C incubator.
3. Aspirate and discard the medium, wash flasks 2× with 10 ml RPMI 1640 medium, and remove adherent cells either by rubber policeman or Trypsin-EDTA treatment.

Comments

1. Some researchers recommend using medium supplemented with 10% FCS, human serum, or autologous human serum.[8]
2. If a sterile cell suspension is required, perform all steps in a laminar flow hood.

4. Removal or purification of monocytes[9]

Materials and reagents

- Cell suspension
- Baby hamster kidney (BHK) cells (ATCC #6281)
- RPMI 1640 medium with 10% FCS
- RPMI 1640 medium with 1% FCS
- PBS
- 75-cm² tissue culture flasks (Corning; Costar)
- 10 m*M* and 3.3 m*M* EDTA in PBS
- Rubber policeman (Corning; Costar)

Protocol

1. Grow baby hamster kidney cells to confluency in RPMI 1640 medium supplemented with 10% FCS.
2. Remove them from the culture flask with 10 m*M* EDTA-PBS and rinse each flask 3× with PBS.

3. Incubate 2 × 10^7 cells (the cell suspension you want to purify) in 10 ml RPMI 1640 medium with 1% FCS in the flask where the BHK cells were cultured. Incubate at 37°C for 60 min.
4. Decant the nonadherent cells (i.e., population depleted of monocytes) and rinse the flask 3× with PBS. Adherent monocytes are removed after a 10-min incubation with 3.3 m*M* EDTA at 37°C by gentle scraping with a rubber policeman.

Comments

1. The baby hamster kidney cell-pretreated tissue culture flasks can be stored in a –30°C freezer for up to 6 months.

5. Removal of monocytes/macrophages using L-leucine methyl ester[10]

Materials and reagents

- Cell suspension
- 1 m*M* L-leucine methyl ester (Sigma)
- RPMI 1640 medium
- RPMI 1640 medium with 10% FCS
- FCS
- 15-ml conical centrifuge tubes

Protocol

1. Incubate 1 × 10^7 cells in serum-free RPMI 1640 medium containing 1 m*M* L-leucine methyl ester. Incubate for 40 min at room temperature.
2. Wash twice in serum-free RPMI 1640 medium by centrifugation at 300*g* for 10 min at 4°C and resuspend in RPMI 1640 medium with 10% FCS.

Comments

1. NK cells and cytotoxic T cells will be also killed.

D. Purification of cell populations using magnetic microspheres

Only recently has magnetic attraction been used to separate cells, although magnetic separators have been used in industry for many years. However, isolation of cells using magnetic synthetic microspheres has recently become more popular. The principle of this technique is quite simple. The cell separation is performed in a liquid phase and is based on the phenomenon that a nonhomogeneous magnetic field can cause small magnetic particles to migrate. Thus, magnetically responsive particles are offered either to phagocytic cells or to any cell suspension. After phagocytosis, phagocytes become magnetized and can be rapidly and gently removed by passing through a nonhomogeneous magnetic field. However, more general methods entail techniques by which the magnetic particles are not necessarily internalized, but only attached to the cell surface. The original technique was described by Molday et al.[14] Their method was very simple; the cells were merely allowed to settle on a column placed near the pole of a permanent magnet. Readers interested in details regarding the preparation of magnetic affinity microspheres should read Reference 15. Recent years, however, have introduced a booming field of commercially available microspheres using an optimal size of particles together with a high-gradient magnetic separation column placed in a strong magnetic field. Using this experimental design, the labeled cells are retained in the column while nonlabeled cells pass through. Subsequently, the column is removed from the magnetic field and the retained cells are eluted. Both fractions (i.e., labeled and nonlabeled), can be recovered.

Several studies prefer different types of microspheres. However, in our hands, the best results were achieved using the Dynabeads. Microspheres from Miltenyi Biotec Inc. are so small that, for most experiments (such as flow cytometry), one does not need to remove the beads from the cells, which substantially speeds up the isolation. These MicroBeads are approximately 50 nm in diameter, which means that they behave more like antibodies, and are biodegradable, which means that positively selected cells can be used for analysis without microsphere removal. In addition to the wide range of microspheres coupled with individual anti-CD antibodies, numerous kits oriented toward depletion of several cell populations in one step are available. In addition, microspheres coupled with FITC, PE, or streptavidin can be purchased. Another interesting possibility represents a MultiSort isolation. The idea is sequential positive selection of cells. Between individual selection steps, microspheres are enzymatically removed. An extremely high enrichment of even very rare cells can be achieved.

A modification of this technique is the use of the new DETACHaBEAD from Dynal, Inc. This product was developed for rapid detachment of cells bound to Dynabeads. DETACHaBEAD is a special polyclonal antibody preparation that reacts with the F(ab) fragments of mouse monoclonal antibodies, subsequently disturbing and blocking the interaction between Dynabeads and the cell surface. The entire technique represents a double magnetic isolation and results in a purified population of the selected cell type (i.e., positive separation). The only disadvantage thus far is the still-limited number of Dynabeads available (the new Dynabeads, specifically designed for use with DETACHaBEAD, are coated with anti-human CD4, CD8, CD19, and CD34 and anti-mouse CD4 only).

In addition to the DETACHaBEAD system, microspheres for both positive and negative selection are available. In addition to beads for immunology, the company offers Dynabeads for cancer research, organelle, protein, and even DNA and RNA.

Materials and reagents

- Magnetic microspheres (Dynal, Inc.; Miltenyi Biotec, Inc.; Advanced Magnetics)
- Cell suspension
- Appropriate monoclonal antibodies (in case microspheres are not directly coupled to antibodies)
- Centrifuge tubes (size according to the type of magnetic device)
- RPMI 1640 medium
- Plastic Pasteur pipettes
- Rotator
- Magnet

Protocol

1. Incubate cells with monoclonal antibodies in centrifuge tube for 30 min at 4°C on a rotator with end-over-end rotation. The most common concentration is 1 g/10^6 cells, but pilot flow cytometry experiments might allow use of even lower concentrations.
2. Wash cells 2× by centrifugation in RPMI 1640 medium at 150*g* at 4°C.
3. Add anti-Ig-coated magnetic microspheres according to manufacturer's instructions and incubate for 60 min at 4°C on a rotator with end-over-end rotation.
4. Separate microsphere-coated cells using the magnetic apparatus. After 5 min, carefully transfer the unbound cells to a new tube using a plastic Pasteur pipette and repeat the magnetic separation.
5. Wash cells 2× by centrifugation in RPMI 1640 medium at 150*g* at 4°C and count them.
6. Before the technique becomes routine (and after using a new batch of antibodies), analyze the isolated cell population by flow cytometry.

Comments

1. This technique can be used for depletion (negative selection) or isolation (positive selection) of any cell subset against which appropriate monoclonal antibodies are available. (Thus, this method is not repeated in individual sections of this chapter).
2. One can combine several monoclonal antibodies in one step; for example, use mouse anti-CD14, mouse anti-CD19, and mouse anti-CD8, and subsequently anti-mouse Ig-coated magnetic microspheres for depletion of monocytes, B cells and $CD8^+$ T cells. The separation will result in pure $CD4^+$ T cells. Check the availability of kits.
3. For best results, repeat isolation steps twice.
4. If a sterile cell suspension is required, perform all steps in a laminar flow hood.

5. Even if optimal results are achieved using magnetic devices available from a company supplying immunobeads, it is not necessary to purchase several, rather expensive types of magnets, as the use of different magnets is only less convenient.
6. Use of directly labeled magnetic beads allows one to skip Steps 1 and 2 and speeds up the entire procedure.

E. *Purification of cells using prepared columns*

Materials and reagents

- RPMI 1640 medium with 5% FCS
- Pipettes
- Separation Cellect column (Biotex)
- Centrifuge tubes
- Cell suspension

Protocol

1. Reconstitute column reagents (provided).
2. Add these reagents to a column and incubate 60 min at room temperature.
3. Add RPMI 1640 medium with 5% FCS and set flow rate according to the manufacturer's instructions.
4. Add cell suspension and incubate for 30 min at room temperature.
5. Add RPMI 1640 medium with 5% FCS and collect enriched cells.

Comments

1. The number of cells per column is different according to the type of column used.
2. At the present time, columns prepared for isolation of human, mouse, and rat T lymphocytes, and CD4 and CD8 lymphocytes are available.

F. *Isolation of resident pulmonary lymphocytes*

Resident peripheral lymphocytes remain in the lung and cannot be removed — even by extensive perfusion of the tissue vascular bed. This technique isolates the cells from the intraepithelial and interstitial spaces without the need for any enzymatic digestion; thus, the cells are suitable for phenotypic and/or functional analysis.

Materials and reagents

- Mice
- Stainless steel mesh

- Scissors
- 21G needle
- 20-ml syringes
- 2-ml syringes
- Sterile Pasteur pipettes
- Glass wool
- Petri dishes
- 15-ml centrifuge tubes
- 50-ml centrifuge tubes
- Avertin (10 g 2,2,2,-tribromoethanol dissolved in 10 ml amyl alcohol)
- Ethanol
- Ficoll-Histopaque (Sigma, Pharmacia)
- Heparin (Sigma)
- PBS without calcium and magnesium
- PBS with EDTA
- Trypan blue
- RPMI 1640 medium supplemented with 10% FCD
- Microscope
- Vortex
- CO_2 incubator (humidified, set at 37°C and 5% CO_2)
- 12-well tissue culture plate

Protocol

(*Note*: All materials and reagents must be sterile and proper aseptic techniques must be used when handling these cells.)

1. Inject the mouse i.p. with 100 U (units) of heparin.
2. After 10 min, inject the mouse i.p. with 0.3 ml avertin (diluted 1:40 in PBS).
3. Wait another 10 min.
4. Immobilize the animal on its back on cutting board (or on paper towel) and soak it with ethanol to reduce the possibility of hair becoming airborne.
5. Make a cut through the skin in the inguinal region. With fingers on both sides of the cut, pull toward the tail and head until the peritoneal wall is sufficiently exposed. Soak the peritoneal wall with ethanol.
6. Lift the base of the sternum and make an incision through the diaphragm. Cut laterally along the diaphragm from the middle to the sides.
7. Cut the thoracic cage open on both sides and remove it.
8. Cut the aorta above the liver.
9. Fill a 20-ml plastic syringe with cold PBS; attach a blunt needle and insert the needle into the right atrium of the heart. Flush 10 ml PBS through the vascular bed of the lung until the lobes turn completely white.

10. Cut the lungs and place the separated lobes in 10 ml PBS in a Petri dish on ice.
11. Rinse the tissue well and transfer into a fresh Petri dish with fresh PBS.
12. Repeat Step 11 three times.
13. Transfer the tissue into a Petri dish with PBS-EDTA, soak for 10 minutes, and cut into 2-mm fragments. Tease the fragments through a stainless steel mesh and rinse with a sterile Pasteur pipette.
14. Transfer the cells into a 15-ml polypropylene tube and centrifuge at 250*g* for 5 min. After centrifugation, two fractions should be visible: cells tightly bound to the lung tissue are in the pellet (iRPL); those that can be mechanically dislodged are in suspension (aRPL).
15. Remove the supernatant, add an equal volume of medium, and centrifuge at 300*g* for 15 min at 4°C.
16. Resuspend in 20 ml medium and carefully layer 5 ml of the suspension over 3 ml Ficoll-Histopaque in a 15-ml polystyrene tube. Centrifuge at 350*g* for 10 min.
17. Collect the cells with a siliconized Pasteur pipette. Dilute the suspension into 20 ml medium and centrifuge at 300*g*.
18. If the iRPL cells are needed, resuspend the pellet from Step 15 in 5 ml PBS-EDTA, vortex, and incubate for 10 min on ice. Centrifuge at 500*g* for 4 min.
19. Repeat Step 18 twice.
20. Resuspend the pellet in 25 ml medium, dilute into a 12-well tissue culture plate, and incubate for 24 hr in a 37°C incubator.
21. Remove the cells from the wells, centrifuge once at 300*g* for 10 min, and count the viable cells.

G. *Isolation of lymphocytes from Peyer's patches*

Peyer's patches are nodular formations of lymphoid tissue along the antimesenteric border of the small intestine. They are comprised of lymphocytes, macrophages, and plasma cells. The enzymatic digestion of the patches is preferred over mechanical dispersion.[16]

Materials and reagents

- Mice
- Siliconized 25-ml glass Erlenmeyer flask
- Stirring bar
- Magnetic stirrer
- 37°C incubator
- 50-ml conical tubes
- Nylon cell strainer (Falcon)
- RPMI 1640 medium
- RPMI 1640 medium with 5% FCS

- Dispase/DNA solution (see Chapter 11)
- PBS without calcium and magnesium, with 5% FCS
- 100-ml beaker
- Gavage needle
- Scissors
- Forceps
- Disposable 10-ml syringes
- 0.15 *M* NaCl
- Ethanol

Protocol

1. Kill mouse, either by cervical dislocation or CO_2 inhalation. Place the mouse on cutting board (or on paper towel) and soak it with ethanol to reduce the possibility of hair becoming airborne.
2. Make a cut through the skin in the inguinal region. With fingers on both sides of the cut, pull toward the tail and head until the peritoneal wall is sufficiently exposed. Soak the peritoneal wall with ethanol.
3. Cut the peritoneal wall and expose the gut. Cut the terminal ileum transversely about 10 mm proximal to the ileocecal junction. Secure the proximal extremity of the section with forceps and gently pull upward while maintaining the mesentery in place with another forceps.
4. Place the gut into the beaker containing 30 ml of 0.15 *M* NaCl. Using the gavage needle attached to the syringe, flush the gut with 10 ml of 0.15 *M* NaCl and place the cleaned gut into the Petri dish. Using the curved scissors, dissect the Peyer's patches.
5. Transfer the Peyer's patches into the Erlenmeyer flask containing 20 ml RPMI and a stirring bar. Gently stir for 10 min at room temperature.
6. Discard the supernatant and repeat Step 5 three times.
7. Replace the washing medium with 10 ml dispase/DNAase solution and gently stir for 30 min at 37°C.
8. Collect the supernatant in a 50-ml conical tube containing 35 ml RPMI with 5% FCS and keep on ice.
9. Repeat Steps 7 and 8 four times.
10. Centrifuge the tubes at 250*g* for 10 min at 4°C. Resuspend and pool the pellets in RPMI with 5% FCS and filter through a nylon cell strainer.

Comments

1. If one needs to use the cells in culture, use only sterile material. Add antibiotics into all media and buffers. Proper aseptic technique must be used when handling these cells.
2. One mouse will yield approximately 1.5×10^7 cells.

H. Isolation of spleen dendritic cells

Dendritic cells are present in most tissues of the body. Based on their characteristics, several types of dendritic cells have been described; for example, veiled cells, interdigitating cells, interstitial dendritic cells follicular dendritic cells, and Langerhans cells. Dendritic cells are of myeloid origin and migrate from the bone marrow via the bloodstream to peripheral tissues. Upon activation, they mature and acquire specific properties. The question as to whether dendritic cells represent a single group of related cells or if they represent a variety of different cell types remains unanswered. At present, at least two distinctive cell types can be identified with heterogeneity apparent in each.[17]

Materials and reagents

- Mice
- 50-ml conical centrifuge tubes
- 15-ml conical centrifuge tubes
- Petri dishes
- 10-ml plastic syringes
- 19-G needles
- Anti-mouse IgG Dynabeads (Dynal) or any similar microbeads
- Water bath
- Humidified incubator
- Scissors
- Forceps
- RPMI 1640 supplemented with 5×10^{-5} *M* mercaptoethanol, glutamine, and antibiotics
- Iscove's medium
- Normal mouse serum, heat inactivated
- Collagenase (Sigma) at 8 mg/ml in medium
- DNAase (Sigma) at 10 mg/ml in PBS
- Percoll (Pharmacia)
- 0.22 μm filter

Protocol

1. Isolate spleens as described above. Cut the spleens into small pieces and transfer into Petri dishes.
2. Prepare 40 ml sterile medium with 1% mouse serum. Keep at room temperature.
3. Prepare 60% Percoll solution and keep at room temperature.
4. Prepare the enzymatic cocktail of 2 ml DNAase, 6 ml collagenase, and 12 ml Iscove's medium. Sterilize through a 0.22-μm filter and keep at 37°C.

5. Make a single-cell suspension of the digested spleen fragments using a 10-ml syringe and 19-G needle. Place the cells into a 50-ml conical tube and fill the tube with Iscove's medium. Wait 2 min so that the debris will settle and transfer the cell suspension into new tubes.
6. Wash 2× by centrifugation at 250*g* for 7 min.
7. Resuspend the cells in 60% Percoll and underlay 5 ml into polystyrene 50-ml tube containing 10 ml Iscove's medium. Centrifuge at 350*g* for 20 min.
8. Harvest the cells from the interface, wash 2× in Iscove's medium, and resuspend in RPMI 1640 medium with 1% mouse serum. Warm for 5 min at 37°C.
9. Place 5 ml cell suspension into 100-mm Petri dish and incubate for 90 min at 37°C. Warm 150 ml RPMI 1640 medium to 37°C. Prepare 20 ml RPMI 1640 with 0.5% mouse serum and warm to 37°C.
10. Wash nonadherent cells from the Petri dishes. Add 5 ml RPMI 1640 with 0.5% mouse serum to each dish and incubate overnight at 37°C. Cells should become nonadherent. Wash the cells 3× by centrifugation at 300*g* at 4°C. As the cells are sticky, coat the tubes with serum.
11. Pool the cells, count them, and resuspend in 3 ml serum-free RPMI 1640 medium on ice.
12. Remove contaminating B lymphocytes with anti-mouse IgG microbeads (as described above).
13. Count the purified cell population.

Comments

1. At Step 10, one can check the dishes using an inverted microscope to ensure that all small, rounded cells have been washed out. The use of the more traditional isolation technique employing BSA density gradient rather than Percoll and FCS instead of mouse serum might result in higher yields of dendritic cells.[18] However, FCS can influence the biological characteristics and properties of dendritic cells.

I. Isolation of peripheral blood cells

1. Ficoll Hypaque separation of neutrophils and mononuclear cells

Materials and reagents

- Peripheral blood
- 3.8% sodium citrate in H_2O
- 50-ml conical centrifuge tubes
- 3% dextran T-500 (Sigma)
- PBS
- Ring stand

- 30-ml disposable syringes
- 18G1 needle
- Tygon tubing 3/32 × 5/32 × 1/32" (Fisher)
- Ficoll-Hypaque/Histopaque
- Plastic transfer pipettes (Fisher)
- PE-160 Intramedic polyethylene tubing

Protocol

1. Draw desired amount of fresh peripheral blood into a syringe containing sodium citrate (5 ml per 60 ml blood).
2. Mix the blood with an equal volume of 3% dextran T-500 in PBS.
3. Draw the mixture into syringes and place the syringe on a ring stand, with the tip facing up. Place Tygon tubing on the tip.
4. Incubate 30 min at room temperature to allow sedimentation of red blood cells.
5. Place the leukocyte-rich plasma into 50-ml centrifuge tubes, 10 to 12 ml per tube.
6. Underlayer the mixture with 12 ml of 1.08 g/ml Ficoll Hypaque using a 30-ml syringe with an 18-gauge needle and PE-160 Intramedic polyethylene tubing.
7. Then, underlayer the first layer with 12 ml of 1.105 g/ml Ficoll-Hypaque.
8. Centrifuge for 30 min at 1000*g* at room temperature.
9. Harvest the cells with a plastic transfer pipette from the two interfaces from each tube: the top white cell layer between the plasma and the 1.08 Ficoll-Hypaque is a mixture of mononuclear cells (lymphocytes and monocytes) and platelets; the bottom layer between the 1.08 and 1.105 Ficoll-Hypaque contains mostly neutrophils.
10. Pool the homologous layers from up to three tubes into a 50-ml conical tube and dilute to full tube capacity with PBS (room temperature).
11. Centrifuge at 400*g* for 12 min at room temperature.
12. Decant and blot the tubes.
13. Resuspend and wash cells at least 2× with PBS, centrifuging at 250*g* for 10 min.
14. Resuspend the cells in the desired media and count.

2. Isolation of basophils

Materials and reagents

- Peripheral blood
- 3.8% sodium citrate in H_2O

- 50-ml conical centrifuge tubes
- 30-ml disposable syringes
- 18G1 needle
- Percoll
- Plastic transfer pipettes
- HBSS without Ca^{2+} and Mg^{2+}
- 0.25 *M* HEPES
- 1 *M* HCl

Protocol

1. Prepare a stock solution by mixing the following:
   a. 90 ml Percoll
   b. 9 ml of 10X HBSS
   c. 1 ml of 0.25 *M* HEPES
   d. 0.4 ml 1 *M* HCl

2. Prepare the following densities of Percoll:
   a. 1.070 g/ml: 24.0 ml Percoll stock mixed with 20.0 ml of 1X HBSS
   b. 1.079 g/ml: 27.0 ml Percoll stock mixed with 15.9 ml of 1X HBSS
   c. 1.088 g/ml: 23.0 ml Percoll stock mixed with 10.0 ml of 1X HBSS

3. Form a Percoll gradient by sequentially adding to the bottom of the tube 4 ml of 1.070 g/ml solution, 4 ml of 1.079 g/ml solution, and 3 ml of 1.088 g/ml solution.
4. Carefully layer 4 ml freshly collected peripheral blood over Percoll gradients and centrifuge 25 min at 300*g* at room temperature with brake off.
5. Collect cells from each cell band with a plastic transfer pipette. Pool same bands from each gradient tube into one 15-ml centrifuge tube. Place 3.3-ml aliquots in new, separate 15-ml tubes.
6. Wash each aliquot 2× with 10 ml of HBSS by centrifugation at 300*g* at 4°C for 10 min.

Comments

1. Basophils are usually found in the middle band; but due to the donor-to-donor variations, check all bands by Giemsa-Wright staining.
2. Peripheral blood basophils are very rare; therefore, this procedure results in 15 to 50% enrichment only (depending on the donor). One can further purify the population using some of the methods mentioned above (such as negative selection of contaminating cells by magnetic microspheres).

References

1. Vetvicka, V., Zeleny, V., and Viklicky, V., Cell surface changes of the mouse peritoneal macrophages after proteose peptone or thioglycollate induction, *Fol. Biol.*, 25, 156, 1979.
2. Fornusek, L., Vetvicka, V., and Kopecek, J., Differences in phagocytic activity of methacrylate copolymer particles in normal and stimulated macrophages, *Experientia*, 37, 418, 1981.
3. Parish, C.R., Kirov, S.M., Bowern, N., Blanden, N., and Blanden, R.V., A one-step procedure for separating mouse T and B lymphocytes, *Eur. J. Immunol.*, 4, 808, 1974.
4. Swain, S.L., Significance of Lyt phenotypes: Lyt2 antibodies block activation of T cells that recognize class I MHC antigens regardless of their function, *Proc. Natl. Acad. Sci. U.S.A.*, 78, 7101, 1981.
5. Wysocki, W.L. and Sato, V.L., "Panning" for lymphocytes: a method for cell selection, *Proc. Natl. Acad. Sci. U.S.A.*, 75, 2844, 1978.
6. Julius, M.H., Simpson, E., and Herzenberg, L.A., A rapid method for the isolation of functional thymus-derived murine lymphocytes, *Eur. J. Immunol.*, 3, 645, 1973.
7. Ly, I.A. and Mishell, R.I., Separation of mouse spleen cells by passage through columns of Sephadex G-10, *J. Immunol. Methods*, 5, 239, 1974.
8. Edelson, P.J. and Cohn, Z.A., Purification and cultivation of monocytes and macrophages, in *In vitro Methods in Cell-mediated and Tumor Immunity*, Bloom, B.A. and Davis, J.R., Eds., Academic Press, San Diego, 1976, 333.
9. Ackerman, S.K. and Douglas, S.D., Purification of human monocytes on microexudate-coated surfaces, *J. Immunol.*, 120, 1372, 1978.
10. Thiele, D.L., Kurosaka, M., and Lipsky, P.E., Phenotype of the accessory cell necessary for mitogen-stimulated T and B cell responses in human peripheral blood: delineation by its sensitivity to the lysosomotropic agent, L-leucine methyl ester, *J. Immunol.*, 131, 2282, 1983.
11. Oda, M. and Puck, T.T., The interaction of mammalian cells with antibodies, *J. Exp. Med.*, 113, 599, 1960.
12. Basch, R.S., Berman, J.W., and Lakow, E., Cell separation using positive immunoselective techniques, *J. Immunol. Methods*, 56, 269, 1983.
13. Vetvicka, V., Fornusek, L., and Tlaskalova, H., Comparison of different methods for separation of human, mouse and rat macrophages and lymphocytes, *Fol. Biol.*, 27, 144, 1981.
14. Molday, R.S., Yen, S.P.S., and Rembaum, A., Application of magnetic microspheres in labeling and separation of cells, *Nature*, 268, 437, 1977.
15. Fornusek, L. and Vetvicka, V., Polymeric microspheres as diagnostic tools for cell surface marker tracing, *CRC Crit. Rev. Therap. Drug Carrier Sys.*, 2, 137, 1986.
16. Frangakis, M.V., Koopman, W.J., Kyono, H., Michalek, S.M., and McGhee, R., An enzymatic method for preparation of dissociated murine Peyer's patch cells enriched for macrophages, *J. Immunol. Meth.*, 48, 33, 1982.

17. Tew, J.G., Burton, G.F., Masuda, A., Kapasi, Z.F., and Szakal, A.K., Dendritic cells as accessory cells, in *Immune System Accessory Cells*, Fornusek, L. and Vetvicka, V., Eds., CRC Press, Boca Raton, FL, 1992, 131.
18. Crowley, M., Inaba, K., Witmer-Pack, M.D., and Steiman, R.M., The cell surface of mouse dendrite cells from different tissues including thymus, *Cell Immunol.*, 118, 108, 1989.

chapter two

Flow cytometry

Contents

I. Overview

The principle of flow cytometry is rather simple: to scan single cells flowing past an excitation source in a liquid medium and analyze them according to their fluorescence. In a typical flow cytometer, a suspension of fluorescently labeled cells is made to flow in a laminar manner by a suitable hydrodynamic system such that they line up in single file. As they move, they cross a beam of light from a laser. As a result, two types of light — scattered light and fluorescent light — are transmitted.

To describe the various techniques used in either cell surface analysis or cell sorting, it would be beneficial to introduce some terminology. The purpose of this chapter is to survey the most commonly used techniques and to either suggest some modifications or to point out some possible pitfalls. To discuss the advantages of one cell cytometer against another or which cell cytometer would be better for your laboratory falls out of the scope of this chapter.

Flow cytometers can have one or more light sources. The most commonly utilized light source is a laser because it exhibits the highest attainable spectral radiance. Readers seeking more details should consult Reference 1. Each light beam is operated at a single wavelength, which will restrict the use of the various probes. Similarly, fluorescence emissions from different probes that excite at a single wavelength will often have spectral overlap (see Table 2.1). Proper understanding of these parameters is essential for determining which fluorescent probes one might employ. A second excitation source significantly expands the availability of probes to be used simultaneously.

Table 2.1 Dyes Commonly Used in Flow Cytometry

Dye	Ex_{min} (nm)	Ex_{max} (nm)	Laser Line (nm)	Emission Range (nm)
DAPI	365	450	351–364	380–420
AO	500	530 (DNA)	488	510–530
AO	500	640 (RNA)	488	590–640
Ethidium	490	610	514, 488	550–640
PI	490	625	514, 488	550–640
FITC	494	517	488	510–530
PE	460	560	488	550–600
RITC	545	600	514	600–620
Lucifer yellow	280–430	540	351–364	500–550
Texas red	595	615	610	620–630
TRITC	460	555	488	530–570
INDO–1	352	450	351–364	400–580
Fura–2	362	340	351–364	300–400
Fluo–3	500	610	488	520–540

The spectral overlap can be compensated using **electronic compensation**. Electronic compensation means subtraction of a percentage of the signal measured from the first probe from that of the second probe. The commonly used fluorochromes — fluorescein isothiocyanate (FITC) and phycoerythrin (PE) — can serve as an example. FITC is measured at a peak of 530 nm as green fluorescence, and PE at a peak of 575 nm as orange fluorescence. However, a significant part of the green fluorescence also appears in the orange emission (and much less of orange in green emission). It is optimal to set the electronic compensation before running the real samples. The easiest way is to mix cells labeled with a single fluorochrome and unlabeled cells, run these cells, and then set the electronic compensation in such a way that the amount of orange (in the case of FITC-labeled cells) fluorescence of positive cells is equal to that of unlabeled cells. The same must be done for cells labeled with PE. However, it is important to note that due to the high possibility of false negativity or false positivity, the use of proper controls (cells stained with only one fluorochrome) for all reagent-cell combinations is often necessary. This is especially true when pairs of fluorochromes with extreme differences in intensity are used.

The **detector voltage** is the voltage used to operate a photomultiplier tube. The level of detector voltage should always be such as to keep both negative and positive cell populations on a histogram.

Forward light scatter (FALS) is measured in front of the path of excitation light and is the detection of the amount of excitation light scattered by a cell in that particular light beam. Both cell refractive index and cell size influence forward light scatter. FALS is proportional to cell size at narrow forward angle. It is more common to use a dual-angle light scatter combination, usually forward-angle light scatter and 90° light scatter.

Gates define the parameters for the cells of interest. On a two-parameter contour histogram, one can draw a box defining the region (cell type) of interest.

Regardless of the detection system, the correct use of optical **filters** is critical. Two types of filters are used: absorbance filters and interference (dichroic) filters. Absorbance filters absorb short wavelengths and pass only long wavelengths. Interference filters, on the other hand, are coated such that they are selective mirrors that block by reflecting certain wavelengths and passing other wavelengths. In practice, both types of filters are used simultaneously to block all unwanted light.

A **bit map** is the part of the contour diagram that has been selected for further study. Thus, the desired (i.e., fluorescence) parameter(s) will be measured for each bit map.

List mode is a form of data storage. This type of storage allows retrospective analysis of stored data, but requires huge storage capacity.

Calibration is the safest way to achieve consistency in day-to-day operation of a flow cytometer. It is important to check the machine by a quick analysis of a sample of fluorescent microspheres for which the coefficient of variation was determined just after the machine was optimally calibrated by a serviceman.

There are many other applications of cell cytometers, such as cell sorting, mitochondrial stains, measurement of intracellular pH, glutathione, membrane fluidity, membrane potential, phagocytosis, virus adsorption, pinocytosis, cell killing, or enzyme analysis. Most of these methods reach far beyond immunology and readers seeking more detailed description of both principles of flow cytometry and all possible applications should read some of the comprehensive reviews.[1-5]

A. *Labeling of antibodies with fluorescein isothiocyanate (FITC)*

Materials and reagents

- Ascites fluid or serum
- $(NH_4)_2SO_4$ or Na_2SO4
- Dimethylsulfoxide (DMSO; Sigma)
- 5 mg/ml FITC in DMSO (prepare fresh before use)
- FITC labeling buffer
- Dialysis buffer
- 5-ml glass tube
- Dialyzing tube

Protocol

1. Purify IgG from monoclonal ascites or serum by $(NH_4)_2SO_4$- or Na_2SO_4-precipitation (see Chapter 10) and dialyze overnight at 4°C against FITC labeling buffer, pH 9.2. Check the concentration ($A_{280} \times 0.74 \times$ Dilution = mg/ml) and adjust it to 1 to 2 mg/ml.
2. Add 20 μl diluted FITC (in a glass tube) per 1 mg of antibody and incubate 2 hr at room temperature.
3. Dialyze the unbound FITC by dialysis against dialysis buffer. Check the concentration and determine the FITC/protein ratio.
4. Measure the optical density at A_{280} and A_{492}.

$$\text{Protein concentration in mg/ml} = A_{280} - (A_{492} \times 0.35)/1.4$$

$$\text{Protein in moles} = \text{Protein mg/ml}/1.5 \times 10^5$$

$$\text{FITC in moles} = A_{492}/0.69 \times 10^5$$

$$\text{FITC/protein ratio} = \text{Moles of FITC/Moles of protein}$$

Comments

1. As an alternative to dialysis, one can remove the unbound FITC by passage through a Sephadex G-25 column.
2. 1.5×10^5 and 0.69×10^5 values in the calculation of the FITC/protein ratio are the molecular weight of immunoglobulin and the molar extinction coefficient of FITC, respectively.
3. The optimal FITC/protein ratio for flow cytometry is usually 2 to 5:1.

B. *Labeling of antibodies with biotin*

Materials and reagents

- Ascites fluid or serum
- $(NH_4)_2SO_4$ or Na_2SO_4
- Dimethylsulfoxide (DMSO) or dimethylformamide (DMF; Fisher)
- NaN_3
- 5-ml glass tube
- Bovine serum albumin (BSA)
- 0.1 *M* $NaHCO_3$, pH 8.5
- D-Biotin-*N*-hydroxysuccinimide ester (BNHS; Boehringer Mannheim #732-494)
- Dialyzing tube

Protocol

1. Purify IgG from monoclonal ascites or serum by $(NH_4)_2SO_4$- or Na_2SO_4-precipitation (see Chapter 10) and dialyze against 0.1 *M* $NaHCO_3$, pH 8.5. Adjust concentration to 1 mg/ml.
2. Dissolve BNHS in DMSO at 1 mg/ml in a glass tube.
3. Add 200 μl of DMSO solution to 800 μl of antibody (250 μg/mg protein) and incubate for 1 hr at room temperature.
4. Dialyze against PBS containing 0.05% of NaN_3 and 0.1% BSA.

C. *Alternate method for biotinylation of antibodies*

Materials and reagents

- D-Biotin-*N*-hydroxysuccinimide ester (BNHS; Boehringer-Mannheim #732-494)
- Dimethylformamide (DMF)
- Glass tube
- Ascites fluid or serum
- $(NH_4)_2SO_4$ or Na_2SO_4
- Borate-buffered saline, pH 8.4 (BBS)
- Dialyzing tube

Protocol

1. Purify IgG from mouse monoclonal ascites by $(NH_4)_2SO_4$- or Na_2SO_4-precipitation (see Chapter 10) and dialyze against BBS (pH 8.43). Adjust concentration to 3 mg/ml.

2. Dissolve BNHS ester in dimethylformamide (1.1 mg BNHS/100 μl DMF) in a **glass** tube.
3. Add 25 μl BNHS/DMF to 0.5 ml antibody (183 μg/mg protein).
4. Incubate 7 hr at room temperature.
5. Dialyze against BBS and render 0.05% in NaN_3.

Comments

1. The entire procedure can be performed in the dialysis tubing. Clamp tubing at first dialysis. Add BNHS directly to dialysis bag, reclamp, and incubate in a moist environment (Petri dish with wet gauze) at room temperature. Redialyze in the same tubing.

D. Labeling antibodies with Texas red

Texas red is a sulfonylchloride derivate of sulforhodamine 101 and is used for double staining.[6]

Materials and reagents

- Texas red labeling buffer (see Chapter 11)
- Texas red (1 mg/ml in cold anhydrous acetonitrile; Sigma)
- Ascites fluid or serum
- $(NH_4)_2SO_4$ or Na_2SO_4
- Dialysis buffer
- 5-ml glass tube
- Dialyzing tube
- Ice
- Spectrofluorimeter

Protocol

1. Purify IgG from monoclonal ascites or serum by $(NH_4)_2SO_4$- or Na_2SO_4-precipitation (see Chapter 10) and dialyze against Texas red labeling buffer. Adjust concentration to 1 mg/ml.
2. Add 100 μl of diluted Texas red per 1 mg of antibody and incubate for 2 hr on ice.
3. Dialyze the unbound Texas red by dialysis against dialysis buffer (Chapter 11).
4. Determine the Texas red/antibody ratio via spectrofluorimetry by measuring A_{596}/A_{280}.

Comments

1. The best results are usually achieved with ratios of 0.7 to 0.9.

E. *Staining of cells for detection of surface antigens*

Materials and reagents

- Cell suspension
- Labeled or unlabeled antibody
- Labeled secondary antibody (in case of unlabeled primary antibody)
- 100 μg/ml propidium iodide
- 5-ml centrifuge tubes
- RPMI 1640 medium with 5% FCS
- Flow cytometer
- Ice

Protocol

1. Put 0.1 ml of cells (1×10^5) into centrifuge tubes.
2. Add 10 μl of appropriately diluted antibody to each tube and incubate for 30 min on ice.
3. Wash the cells 2× by centrifugation at 300*g* for 10 min on ice. Discard supernatant and resuspend cell pellet in 0.1 ml cold RPMI 1640 medium with 5% FCS.
4. In case of unlabeled primary antibodies, repeat Steps 2 and 3 with labeled secondary antibodies.
5. Run the samples on the flow cytometer.

Comments

1. Add 10 μl of diluted propidium iodide simultaneously with last antibody.
2. Do not use propidium iodide with antibodies labeled with phycoerythrin.
3. Always use a negative control. The adequate negative control is either an irrelevant antibody of the same isotype as antibody used (for direct labeling) or secondary labeled antibody only.
4. Centrifuge all antibodies at 10,000*g* for 20 min prior to use in order to remove all aggregates.

F. *Staining of cells for detection of surface antigens in plates*[7]

Materials and reagents

- Cell suspension
- Labeled or unlabeled antibody
- Labeled secondary antibody (in case of unlabeled primary antibody)
- 100 μg/ml propidium iodide
- 96-well, round-bottom microtiter plates (Costar)

- RPMI 1640 medium with 5% FCS
- Flow cytometer
- BSA
- PBS
- NaN_3
- Ice

Protocol

1. Prepare PBS supplemented with 12% BSA and 10 m*M* NaN3 (12% BSA/PBS/azide).
2. Put 0.1 ml of cells (1×10^5 cells/well) into wells of a 96-well plate.
3. Add 10 µl of appropriately diluted antibody to each well, mix, and incubate for 30 min on ice.
4. Wash the cells once by centrifugation through a 0.1-ml cushion of 12% BSA/PBS/azide.
5. In case of unlabeled primary antibodies, repeat Steps 2 and 3 with labeled secondary antibodies.
6. Wash the cells once by centrifugation through a 0.1-ml cushion of 12% BSA/PBS/azide.
7. Run the samples on the flow cytometer.

Comments

1. Add 10 µl diluted propidium iodide simultaneously with last antibody.
2. Do not use propidium iodide with antibodies labeled with phycoerythrin.
3. Always use a negative control. The adequate negative control is either an irrelevant antibody of the same isotype as antibody used (for direct labeling) or secondary labeled antibody only.
4. Centrifuge all antibodies at 10,000*g* for 20 min prior to use in order to remove all complexes.
5. Use this modification only when a large number of samples is to be tested.

G. *Detection of intracellular antigens*

This technique can be used either for intracellular staining alone or for combined simultaneous staining of surface and internal antigens. In such a case, cells that have been labeled for cell surface expression using one fluorescent dye can also be labeled for expression of intracellular antigens using a second fluorescent dye.[8-11] The combination of two fluorescent dyes is not relevant as long as the excitation spectra are distinguishable; the only limitation is the fact that Peridin Chlorophyll Protein (PerCP) cannot be used because its fluorescence is lost after permeabilization.

Materials and reagents

- Cells
- PBS
- Labeled or unlabeled antibody
- Labeled secondary antibody (in case of unlabeled primary antibody)
- 4% paraformaldehyde (Sigma)
- 5-ml tubes
- 0.3% saponin (Sigma) in PBS
- 0.3% saponin in PBS with 10 μl propidium iodide (if you plan to measure DNA content)
- Second labeled antibody (for intracellular staining)
- Ice

Protocol

1. Put 0.1 ml cells (1×10^5) into centrifuge tubes.
2. Dilute the labeled antibody in PBS containing 0.3% saponin.
3. Add 0.1 ml diluted labeled antibody to the cell suspension, gently mix, and incubate for 30 min at 4°C.
4. Wash the cells 2× by centrifugation at 300*g* for 10 min on ice in PBS. Discard supernatant and resuspend cell pellet in 0.1 ml cold PBS.
5. Fix the cells with 0.1 ml of 4% paraformaldehyde for 20 min on ice.
6. Permeabilize the cells with two washes in PBS containing 0.3% saponin.
7. Add 0.1 ml of second labeled antibody to the cell suspension, gently mix, and incubate for 30 min at 4°C.
8. Wash the cells 2× by centrifugation at 300*g* for 10 min on ice in PBS containing 0.3% saponin. Discard supernatant and resuspend cell pellet in 0.1 ml cold PBS containing 0.3% saponin.
9. Run on flow cytometer.

Comments

1. If the cell membrane has been stained with unlabeled antibody, Steps 3 and 4 must be repeated with labeled secondary antibody.
2. Saponin needs to be present during incubation with second antibody and during all subsequent washings.

3. Alternatively, the technique originally developed for immunofluorescent staining of intracellular cytokines employing intracellular transport inhibitors such as monensin or brefeldin A might be used.[12]

H. *Influx of Ca^{2+} ions using Fluo-3*

The role of Ca^{2+} as an intracellular regulator has attracted a great deal of interest in recent years. Under normal conditions, intracellular free Ca^{2+} concentrations are maintained by ATPase-Ca^{2+} pumps localized in the plasma membrane that keep molarity concentrations far below that of the external media. Healthy cells maintain an intracellular level of free Ca^{2+} about 10,000 times lower than the extracellular environment.

Measurements of the intracellular Ca^{2+} have been important for elucidation of the central role of Ca^{2+}_i as a trigger of the cellular response to activation.

Materials and reagents

- Flow cytometer
- Cells
- RPMI 1640 medium
- Dimethylsulfoxide (DMSO)
- Fluo-3 (Molecular Probes)
- Water bath with cover
- $CaCl_2$
- PBS
- 5-ml plastic disposable tubes with cap

Protocol

1. Wash cells 3× in PBS by centrifugation at 250*g* for 5 min at room temperature.
2. Resuspend cells in RPMI 1640 medium to a final concentration of 5×10^6 cells/ml.
3. Dissolve one tube of the Fluo-3 in 50 μl DMSO.
4. Add 10 μl of the dissolved dye to 140 μl RPMI 1640 medium and mix.
5. Add 90 μl diluted Fluo-3 dye to each milliliter of cell suspension and mix gently.
6. Incubate the mixture of cells and stain for 45 min at 37°C in the dark.
7. Remove 100 μl of suspension and add 400 μl RPMI 1640 medium supplemented with 1 m*M* $CaCl_2$. Incubate for 2 min at 37°C in the dark before adding the test substance.
8. Run the samples on the flow cytometer.

Comments

1. This method can be performed using a single-laser (i.e., argon 488 nm) flow cytometer without any special filters.
2. Do not forget to measure cell suspension before adding the test substance to obtain background levels of Ca^{2+}.

I. *Influx of Ca^{2+} ions using Indo-1*

Materials and reagents

- Flow cytometer
- Cells
- Hanks' balanced salt solution with calcium and magnesium
- Dimethylsulfoxide (DMSO)
- 2 mg/ml Indo-1 pentaacetoxymethyl ester (Indo-1; dissolved in DMSO; Molecular Probes)
- 1 mg/ml ionomycin (dissolved in DMSO; Calbiochem)
- Water bath
- PBS
- Calcium-EGTA buffers
- 5-ml plastic disposable tubes with cap

Protocol

1. Prepare cell suspension and resuspend cells in Hanks' balanced salt solution with calcium and magnesium to a density of 10^6/ml.
2. Put cells into the tubes and add 2 mg/ml Indo-1 solution to a final concentration of 2 μg/ml. Incubate 30 min at 37°C.
3. Centrifuge cells at 200*g* for 10 min at room temperature. Gently resuspend the cells in Hanks' balanced salt solution with calcium and magnesium and incubate for 15 min at room temperature in the dark.
4. Set up the flow cytometer. Use 395-nm and 500-nm bandpass filters.
5. Resuspend cells in a series of calcium-EGTA buffers and ionomycin.[13]
6. Warm an aliquot of Indo-1-loaded cells for 10 min at 37°C. Use 1×10^5 cells per time interval.
7. Analyze cells in flow cytometer. Keep the cells at all times at 37°C.

J. *The respiratory burst of neutrophils*[14]

The respiratory burst is a burst of oxidative metabolic activity associated with the recognition and ingestion of opsonized particles by neutrophils.[15,16] This burst can be also induced by various mediators such as phorbol myristate acetate or N-formyl-methionyl-leucyl-phenylalanine, and is considered to be a sign of functional activation of neutrophils. It is initiated through the stimulation of NADPH oxidase, which catalyzes the transfer of electrons from NADPH to oxygen.[16,17] The flow cytometric measurement of respiratory burst activity is done using the nonfluorescent probe 2′,7′-dichlorofluorescein (DCFH)[18] or diacetyl-2′,7′-dichlorofluorescein (DCFH-DA)[19] which during the respiratory burst are oxidized to the intensely fluorescent 2′,7′-dichlorofluorescein. In addition, dihydrorhodamine 123 is also used. The basis for this type of evaluation of the formation of superoxide and hydrogen peroxide is the theory that these probes remain intracellular as a result of cleavage of ester bonds by cellular esterases.[18] This fact eliminates the possible issue of whether activated probes might be missed owing to diffusion out of the cells. Thus, the cells might be preloaded with the probe and stimulated later.[20]

Materials and reagents

- Freshly isolated neutrophils (see Chapter 1)
- Ethanol
- Diacetyl-2′,7′-dichlorofluorescein (Eastman-Kodak)
- Phorbol myristate acetate (PMA; Sigma)
- DMSO
- 10-ml polystyrene tubes
- Water bath with cover
- Flow cytometer
- Hanks′ balanced salt solution (HBSS)

Protocol

1. Isolate neutrophils and dilute them in Hanks′ balanced salt solution to a concentration of 10^7 cells/ml.
2. Incubate the neutrophils in 5 μ*M* DCFH-DA (prepared from 500 μ*M* stock in ethanol) in 10-ml polystyrene tubes for 15 min at 37°C in the dark.
3. Wash the cells once in Hanks′ balanced salt solution by centrifugation at 250 × *g* for 5 min at room temperature and add 100 μl of appropriate dilution of PMA (from stock solution of 1 mg/ml in DMSO). The optimal concentration of PMA is 50 to 100 ng/ml. Incubate for 15 min at 37°C in the dark.
4. Place the tube with cells on ice and, without washing, examine the fluorescence using the flow cytometer.

Comments

1. Stock solution of DCFH-DA can be stored at –20°C for 6 months, and the stock solution of PMA at –80°C for 6 months.
2. Use a flow cytometer equipped with a laser providing excitation at 488 nm.
3. PMA is used as a positive control.

K. Alternative technique using DCHF-DA

Materials and reagents

- Freshly isolated neutrophils (see Chapter 1)
- Dichlorodihydrofluorescein diacetate (DCHF-DA; Molecular Probes)
- 10-ml polystyrene tubes
- Water bath with cover
- Flow cytometer
- Hanks' balanced salt solution (HBSS)

Protocol

1. Isolate neutrophils and dilute them in Hanks' balanced salt solution to a concentration of 5×10^6 cells/ml.
2. Incubate 100 µl of neutrophils with 100 µl DCHF-DA (1 µg/ml) in 10-ml polystyrene tubes for 10 min at 37°C in the dark.
3. Place the tube with cells on ice and, without washing, examine the fluorescence using the flow cytometer.

Comments

1. Intracellular fluorescence of DCHF-DA usually changes with time and/or temperature; negative controls are thus extremely important. In addition, labeling the cells in small batches is advisable.

L. H_2O_2 production measurement using dihydrorhodamine 123[21]

Materials and reagents

- Freshly isolated neutrophils (see Chapter 1)
- Dihydrorhodamine 123 (Molecular Probes)
- Propidium iodide
- 10-ml centrifuge tubes
- Flow cytometer
- PMA
- Hanks' balanced salt solution with 10 m*M* HEPES
- Dimethylformamide (DMF)
- PBS

Protocol

1. Incubate 20 µl of cells (2×10^7 cells/ml) with 10 µl dihydrorhodamine 123 solution (1:10 dilution of stock in Hanks' balanced salt solution with 10 m*M* HEPES; stock is 346 µg/ml of dimethylformamide) and 1 ml Hanks balanced salt solution with 10 m*M* HEPES.

2. Incubate for 5 min at 37°C.
3. Add 10 μl PMA (to a final concentration 100 n*M*) to a positive control tube. Continue incubation. Add 5 μl propidium iodide (1 mg/ml in PBS) to counterstain dead cells.
4. Take 250-μl aliquots at 5, 10, and 15 min of incubation.
5. Use a flow cytometer equipped with an argon ion laser providing excitation at 488 nm.

Comments

1. The intracellular oxidization of the nonfluorescent dihydrorhodamine 123 to a green fluorescent rhodamine 123 is a hydrogen peroxide-dependent reaction.

M. Lactoferrin assay[14,22]

This assay measures release of lactoferrin from granules as a function of neutrophil activation.

Materials and reagents

- Freshly isolated neutrophils (see Chapter 1)
- Hanks' balanced salt solution with Ca^{2+}, Mg^{2+}, and 1% BSA (HBSS/1% BSA)
- PBS with 0.1% BSA
- 4% paraformaldehyde in PBS
- Anti-human lactoferrin F(ab) conjugated with FITC (Nordic Immunological)
- PMA
- Flow cytometer
- Eppendorf centrifuge tubes
- 15-ml conical centrifuge tubes

Protocol

1. Resuspend freshly isolated neutrophils at 1×10^6 cells/ml in HBSS/1% BSA and put the suspension on ice.
2. Warm cells at 37°C for 10 min.
3. Put 50 μl of PMA (100 n*M*) as a positive control and 50 μl of tested substance into the appropriate Eppendorf centrifuge tubes and warm for 5 min at 37°C.
4. Add 450 μl cells to each tube, mix, and incubate at 37°C for 10 min.
5. Add 500 μl of 4% paraformaldehyde, mix, and incubate for 20 min at room temperature. Wash once by centrifugation at 500*g* for 5 min at 4°C with ice-cold PBS with 0.1% BSA.
6. Resuspend cells in 45 μl ice-cold PBS with 0.1% BSA.

7. Add 5 μl diluted anti-lactoferrin antibody, mix, and incubate for 30 min at 4°C.
8. Wash 2× by centrifugation at 500*g* for 5 min at 4°C with ice-cold PBS with 0.1% BSA. Resuspend in 500 μl ice-cold PBS with 0.1% BSA.
9. Add 150 μl of 4% paraformaldehyde.
10. Run on flow cytometer equipped with an argon ion laser providing excitation at 488 nm.

N. DNA cell cycle analysis using propidium iodide[2,23]

Materials and reagents

- Propidium iodide solution
- Cell suspension
- 5-ml centrifuge tubes
- RNAse (Sigma)
- Nonidet P-40 (Sigma)
- PBS
- Flow cytometer
- Ice

Protocol

1. Resuspend 1×10^6 cells/ml in PBS with 50 μg/ml propidium iodide solution. Remove 1 ml of this solution to another tube. Add 1 ml propidium iodide solution to the second tube.
2. Incubate for 30 min at 4°C
3. Read on flow cytometer at 488 nm.

Comments

1. Propidium iodide intercalates into double-stranded nucleic acids and is excited by 488-nm lasers.
2. RNAse A degrades double-stranded RNA so the only double-stranded nucleic acid left for binding of propidium iodine is DNA.
3. Propidium iodine is a potential carcinogen. Extreme care when handling is recommended.

O. Alternate method for DNA cell cycle analysis using propidium iodide[23]

Materials and reagents

- Propidium iodide solution
- Cell suspension
- 5-ml centrifuge tubes

- Flow cytometer
- 0.1% sodium citrate

Protocol

1. Mix 1×10^6 cells with 1 ml propidium iodide solution (5 μg/ml of 0.1% sodium citrate) and incubate for 5 min at 4°C.
2. Read on flow cytometer at 488 nm.

Comments

1. Propidium iodide intercalates into double-stranded nucleic acids and is excited by 488-nm lasers.
2. Propidium iodine is a potential carcinogen. Extreme care when handling is recommended.

P. DNA cell cycle analysis using mithramycin[24]

Materials and reagents

- Flow cytometer
- Mithramycin (Sigma)
- Ethanol
- $MgCl_2 \cdot 6H_2O$
- 5-ml centrifuge tubes
- Cell suspension

Protocol

1. Resuspend 1×10^6 cells in 1 ml of 25% ethanol containing 100 μg/ml mithramycin and 15 m*M* $MgCl_2$.
2. Incubate on ice for 20 min.
3. Read on flow cytometer equipped with an argon ion laser at 488 nm. Use the filter for phycoerythrin.

References

1. Wood, J.C.S., Horton, A.F., Byrne, J.D., Pedroso, R.I., Bisnow, M., and Auer, R.E., Dual laser excitation flow cytometry: the state-of-the-art, in *Flow Cytometry: Advanced Research and Clinical Applications*, Vol. 1, Yen, A., Ed., CRC Press, Boca Raton, FL, 1989, 5.
2. Robinson, J.P., Ed., *Handbook of Flow Cytometry Methods*, Wiley-Liss, New York, 1993.
3. Melamed, M.R., Lindomo, T., and Mendelson, M.L., Eds., *Flow Cytometry and Sorting*, 2nd ed., Wiley-Liss, New York, 1990.

4. June, C.H. and Rabinovitch, P.S., Immunofluorescence and cell sorting, in *Current Protocols in Immunology*, Coligan, J.E., Kruisbeek, A.M., Margulies, D.H., Shevach, E.M., and Strober, W., Eds., Greene Publishing and Wiley InterScience, New York, 1991, 5.0.1.
5. McLean Grogan, W. and Collins, J.M., *Guide to Flow Cytometry Methods*, Marcel Dekker, New York, 1990.
6. Titus, J.A., Haugland, R., Sharrow, S.O., and Segal, D.M., Texas red, a hydrophilic, red-emitting fluorophore for use with fluorescein in dual parameter flow microfluorometric and fluorescence microscopic studies, *J. Immunol. Meth.*, 50, 193, 1982.
7. Muto, S., Vetvicka, V., and Ross, G.D., CR3 (CD11b/CD18) expressed by cytotoxic T cells and NK cells is upregulated in a manner similar to neutrophils following stimulation with various activating agents, *J. Clin. Immunol.*, 13, 175, 1993.
8. Jaccoberger, J.W., Cell cycle expression of nuclear proteins, in *Flow Cytometry: Advanced Research and Clinical Application*, Vol. 1, Yen, A., Ed., CRC Press, Boca Raton, FL, 1989, 305.
9. Jacob, M.C., Favre, M., and Bensa, J.C., Membrane cell permeabilization with saponin and multiparametric analysis by flow cytometry, *Cytometry*, 12, 550, 1991.
10. Clevenger, C.V. and Shankey, T.V., Cytochemistry II: Immunofluorescence measurements of intracellular antigens, in *Clinical Flow Cytometry*, Bauer, K.D., Duque, R.E., and Shankey, T.V., Eds., Williams and Wilkins, Baltimore, 1993, 157.
11. Holmes, K., Fowlknes, B.J., Schmid, I., and Giorgi, J.V., Preparation of cells and reagents for flow cytometry, in *Current Protocols in Immunology*, Coligan, J.E., Kruisbeek, A.M., Margulies, D.H., Shevach, E.M., and Strober, W., Eds., Greene Publishing and Wiley InterScience, New York, 1999, 5.3.1.
12. Vetvicka, V., Vetvickova, J., Hilgert, I., Voburka, Z., and Fusek, M., Analysis of the interaction of procathepsin D activation peptide with breast cancer cells, *Int. J. Cancer*, 73, 402, 1997.
13. Chused, T.M., Wilson, H.A., Greenblatt, D., Ishida, Y., Edison, L.J., Tsien, R.Y., and Finkelman, F.D., Flow cytometric analysis of murine splenic B lymphocyte cytosolic free calcium response to anti-IgM and anti-IgD, *Cytometry*, 8, 396, 1987.
14. Kenny, P.A. and Finlay-Jones, J.J., Flow-cytometric measurement of respiratory burst activity of neutrophils, in *Laboratory Methods in Immunology*, Zola, H., Ed., CRC Press, Boca Raton, FL, 1990, 131.
15. Babior, B.M., Oxygen-dependent microbial killing by phagocytes, *N. Engl. J. Med.*, 298, 659, 1978.
16. Rossi, F., Dri, P., Bellavite, P., Zabucchi, G., and Berton, G., Oxidative metabolism of inflammatory cells, *Adv. Inflammation Res.*, 1, 139, 1979.
17. Forman, H.J. and Thomas, M.J., Oxidant production and bactericidal activity of phagocytes, *Annu. Rev. Physiol.*, 48, 669, 1986.
18. Bass, D.A., Parce, J.W., DeChatelet, L.R., Szejda, P., Seeds, P., Seeds, M. C., and Thomas, M., Flow cytometric studies of oxidative product formation by neutrophils: a grade response to membrane stimulation, *J. Immunol.*, 130, 1910, 1983.
19. Brandt, R. and Keston, A.S., Synthesis of diacetyldichlorofluorescein: a stable reagent for fluorimetric analysis, *Anal. Biochem.*, 11, 6, 1965.

20. Stewart, C.C., Multiparameter flow cytometry, *J. Immunoassays*, 21, 255, 2000.
21. Rothe, G., Emmendorffer, A., Oser, A., Roesler, J., and Valet, G., Flow cytometric measurement of the respiratory burst activity of phagocytes using dihydrorhodamine 123, *J. Immunol. Methods*, 128, 133, 1991.
22. Butler, T.W., Heck, L.W., Huster, W.J., Grossi, C.E., and Barton, J.C., Assesment of total immunoreactive lactoferrin in hematopoietic cells using flow cytometry, *J. Immunol. Methods*, 108, 159, 1988.
23. Krishan, A., Rapid flow cytometric analysis of mammalian cell cycle by propidium iodide staining, *J. Cell. Biol.*, 66, 188, 1975.
24. Tobey, R.A. and Crissman, H.A., Unique techniques for cell cycle analysis utilizing mitramycin and flow microfluorometry, *Exp. Cell Res.*, 93, 235, 1975.

chapter three

Proliferation assays

Contents

The assessment of cellular proliferation is perhaps one of the most often used techniques in cellular immunology. Mitogenic activation or specific recognition of antigen by lymphocytes results in the elicitation of a sequence of events that culminate with entry of the cells into cycle and cell division. In addition, preactivated lymphocytes or a variety of cell lines are able to respond to growth-promoting cytokines with increased proliferation.

Because of its simplicity, the measurement of cellular proliferation is routinely used as a convenient way to determine:

1. The magnitude of lymphocytic responses to antigens and/or mitogens
2. The production and concentration of growth-promoting cytokines (bioassays)
3. Cellular toxicity

Although cellular proliferation can be assessed by determining the increase in viable cell numbers through the actual enumeration of cells by direct microscopy or automated cell counting, this approach can be time-consuming, especially when working with a large number of samples or with mixed-cell cultures. Instead, the two most commonly used techniques for the purpose of measuring cellular proliferation are:

- Incorporation of tritiated [^{3}H] thymidine into newly synthesized DNA
- Reduction of tetrazolium dyes, such as 3-[4,5-dimethylthiazol-2-yl]-2,5-diphenyl tetrazolium bromide (MTT), by active mitochondria

These two assays are described below.

I. Incorporation of tritiated thymidine into DNA

As cells enter the "S" phase of the cell cycle, chromosome replication takes place, with the incorporation of soluble nucleotide precursors into newly synthesized DNA. In this assay, dividing cells are incubated ("pulsed") with radioactive [^{3}H] thymidine for several hours, after which the amount of radioactivity incorporated into their DNA is determined by harvesting the cells onto glass fiber filters followed by liquid scintillation counting.

Materials and reagents

- Cells (primary culture, indicator cell lines, etc.)
- Culture medium (depending on the cell culture; for many applications, the culture medium of choice is the RPMI 1640 medium supplemented with 10% FCS, 100 U/ml penicillin, 100 µg/ml streptomycin, 2 m*M* L-glutamine and 50 µ*M* 2-mercaptoethanol)
- [^{3}H-methyl]thymidine (approx. 20 to 50 Ci/mmol), sterile (e.g., Amersham Pharmacia Biotech, NEN Life Science Products)
- 96-well tissue culture plates (flat bottom)
- CO_2 incubator (humidified, set at 37°C and 5% CO_2)
- Multichannel pipette or repeating dispenser
- Cell harvester (Skatron Instruments)
- Glass fiber filter mats (Skatron Instruments)
- Liquid scintillation vials (Research Products International)
- Liquid scintillation cocktail (e.g., Econo-Safe™, Research Products International)
- Liquid scintillation counter

Protocol

1. Plate the indicator cells in 96-well plates in a final volume of 0.1 to 0.2 ml. Usually, each culture condition (e.g., dilution) is tested in triplicate. Include a background proliferation control in which the cells are cultured with medium alone. Incubate at 37°C in a CO_2 incubator for the appropriate length of time.
2. Dilute the [^{3}H-methyl]thymidine stock solution with culture medium to a concentration of 50 µCi/ml. With the aid of a multichannel pipette, add 20 µl of the diluted solution to each well. This gives a final concentration of 1 µCi per well.
3. Return the plates to the incubator. Incubate for an additional 4 to 18 hr. (With rapidly dividing cells, a 4- to 6-hr "pulse" gives adequate results.)
4. Harvest the cells onto glass fiber mats using a cell harvester and distilled water.
5. Allow the filters to air-dry. Place individual filters into liquid scintillation vials and add 2 to 3 ml liquid scintillation cocktail.

6. Count in liquid scintillation counter. Express proliferation data based on cpm or dpm per culture. Alternatively, proliferation data can be expressed as the "Stimulation Index," calculated by dividing the proliferation of the stimulated cells (in cpm) by the background proliferation (in cpm).

Comments

1. The culture medium, the final cell density, and the length of incubation will depend on the nature of the indicator cells and on the nature of the stimulus. Generally, for indicator cell lines that divide rapidly (e.g., HT-2, CTLL), cell densities of 0.5 to 1 × 10^5/ml give adequate results. Freshly isolated lymphocytes or mononuclear cells, on the other hand, require higher cell densities (0.5 to 2 × 10^6/ml). As for incubation times, measurement of proliferation of indicator cell lines to growth-promoting cytokines requires incubations of no more than 48 hr, whereas proliferation of lymphocytes to antigens or mitogens may require incubations as long as 72 to 96 hr.
2. It is important to use tritiated thymidine of high purity and the correct specific activity. It is recommended to use thymidine labeled in the 5-methyl position to avoid the potential risk of labeling RNA due to conversion of thymidine into uridine by demethylation. [^{3}H-methyl]thymidine is commercially available at various specific activities, ranging from 2 to 100 Ci/mmol. The preparations with the lower specific activities are available sterile, in aqueous solution. Ethanol, however, is usually added to the preparations of higher specific activity as a free radical scavenger to reduce radiation decomposition. When using these preparations, one should be aware of the final ethanol concentration, as it may be toxic to some cells.
3. Many liquid scintillation formulations are adequate for this purpose; however, because of the relatively large quantities of radioactive waste generated, the use of a biodegradable liquid scintillation cocktail is recommended.
4. Disintegrations per minute (dpm) = Counts per minute (cpm) ÷ Counting efficiency

II. Nonradioactive detection methods (MTT assay)

Due to the potential hazards associated with the use of radioactive substances, many investigators prefer the use of nonradioactive detection methods for the measurement of cellular proliferation. The most common of these methods is known as the MTT assay.[1] This technique is based on the cleavage of a yellow tetrazolium dye (3-[4,5-dimethylthiazol-2-yl]-2,5-diphenyltetrazolium bromide, MTT) into insoluble purple formazan by dehydrogenases in active mitochondria. Dead cells are unable to perform this reaction. In this assay, an MTT solution is added to the dividing cells and, after a 4-hr incubation period, the amount of purple formazan generated is spectrophotometrically determined using a multiwell spectrophotometer or ELISA reader.

Materials and reagents

- Cells (primary culture, indicator cell lines, etc.)
- Culture medium (depends on the cell culture; for many applications, the culture medium of choice is RPMI 1640 medium supplemented with 10% FCS, 100 U/ml penicillin, 100 μg/ml streptomycin, 2 m*M* L-glutamine, and 50 μ*M* 2-mercaptoethanol)
- 96-well tissue culture plates (flat bottom)
- CO_2 incubator (humidified, set at 37°C and 5% CO_2)
- Multichannel pipette or repeating dispenser
- MTT (Sigma Cat. No. M-5655). Prepare a stock solution of MTT (5 mg/ml) in PBS
- Filter
- Acidic isopropanol (0.04 *N* HCl in isopropanol)
- Multiwell spectrophotometer (ELISA reader)

Protocol

1. Plate the cells in 96-well tissue culture plates as described in the previous chapter section, including cells cultured in medium alone as a background proliferation control (triplicates are recommended). Culture in a CO_2 incubator at 37°C for the appropriate length of time.
2. Using a multichannel pipette, add 10 μl of the MTT stock solution per 100 μl culture medium. (Final MTT concentration is 0.5 mg/ml.)
3. Incubate at 37°C for 4 hr.
4. If the cells are nonadherent, add 100 μl/well of the acidic isopropanol solution directly onto the wells. If the cells are adherent, the medium can be discarded first and then the acidic isopropanol (100 μl per well) can be added directly onto the cells.
5. Mix well and incubate at room temperature until all crystals are dissolved (5 to 10 min).
6. Read on a multiwell spectrophotometer using a test wavelength of 570 nm and a reference wavelength of 630 nm. Read plates within 1 hr of addition of the acidic isopropanol.

Comments

1. Red blood cells do not cleave MTT to a significant extent, nor do they interfere with the assay up to concentrations of 2×10^6 cells/ml.[1]
2. Several modifications to the original assay described by Mosmann[1] have been reported. Most of these modifications address the problem

of protein precipitation, especially when using culture medium containing high serum concentrations during the formazan-extraction step using acidic isopropanol.[2] Sodium dodecyl sulfate (SDS) appears to minimize protein precipitation but requires longer extraction times, whereas isopropanol accelerates the extraction but leads to increased development of turbidity due to protein precipitation. Extraction reagents in some of these modifications include[2]:

a. 10% SDS buffered to pH 4.7 with acetate buffer
b. 10% SDS/50% isopropanol/0.01 *N* HCl, pH 5.5
c. 20% SDS in 50% *N,N*-dimethylformamide buffered to pH 4.7 with acetic acid
d. 3% SDS in acidified (0.04 N HCl) isopropanol

In another modification resulting in improved sensitivity and reproducibility,[3] the normal medium is removed before the addition of MTT. The incubation with MTT is then carried out in serum-free medium devoid of phenol red, thus avoiding the potential precipitation of proteins and the need for acidification. The purple formazan product is then dissolved using propanol or ethanol. This assay uses 560 and 690 nm as the test and reference wavelengths, respectively.

3. Another nonradioactive detection assay for cell proliferation is available from Amersham Pharmacia Biotech. This assay is based on the incorporation of 5-bromo-2′-deoxyuridine (BrdU), a thymidine analog, into DNA, followed by detection of incorporated BrdU using a specific peroxidase-labeled monoclonal antibody against BrdU. This assay is carried out in an ELISA format and is reported to be more sensitive than the traditional [^{3}H]-thymidine incorporation assay.

References

1. Mosmann, T., Rapid colorimetric assay for cellular growth and survival: application to proliferation and cytotoxicity assays, *J. Immunol. Methods*, 65, 55, 1983.
2. Niks, M. and Otto, M., Towards an optimized MTT assay, *J. Immunol. Methods*, 130, 149, 1990.
3. Denizot, F. and Lang, R., Rapid colorimetric assay for cell growth and survival. Modifications to the tetrazolium dye procedure giving improved sensitivity and reliability, *J. Immunol. Methods*, 89, 271, 1986.

chapter four

Preparation of cell clones

Contents

I. Preparation of mouse T cell clones

A. Th clones reactive with soluble antigens[1]

Antigen-specific T cells can usually be cloned into two distinct populations of Th cells: Th1 cells (which produce IL-2 and IFNγ) and Th2 cells (which produce IL-4 and whose proliferation is inhibited by IFNγ).[2] The addition of either ConA-supernatant (containing high levels of IL-2) or MLC-supernatant (containing IL-2, IL-4, and IFNγ) during the cloning process results in the preferential isolation of Th2 or Th1 clones, respectively.

Materials and reagents

- Mice
- Antigen
- Freund's complete adjuvant (Sigma)
- PBS
- DMEM medium with 5% FCS, antibiotics
- Irradiated syngeneic spleen cells
- ConA-supernatant or MLC-supernatant (see Sections B.1 and B.2)
- 96-well, flat-bottom tissue culture plates
- 24-well, flat-bottom tissue culture plates
- Human rIL-2
- Mouse rIFNγ
- Humidified 37°C, 5% CO_2 incubator

Protocol

1. Inject mice subcutaneously with a 1:1 emulsion of antigen (50 μg/ml to 1000 μg/ml) in PBS and Freund's complete adjuvant into both hind foot pads and the base of the tail.
2. Seven days later, remove popliteal, periaortic, and inguinal lymph nodes and spleen (see Chapter 1) and prepare single-cell suspension of lymph node cells and spleen cells. Wash the cells 2× by centrifugation at 350*g* at 4°C in complete medium and count them.
3. Irradiate (2000 to 4000 rad) spleen cells.
4. Culture 2×10^6 lymph node cells for 8 days with 6×10^6 irradiated syngeneic spleen cells with antigen (50 μg/ml to 500 μg/ml) in 1.5 ml complete DMEM medium in each well of a 24-well plate in a humidified 37°C, 5% CO_2 incubator.
5. Add the following to each well of a 96-well flat-bottom tissue culture plate:
   50 μl irradiated syngeneic spleen cells (2×10^7 cells/ml)
   50 μl antigen (200 μg/ml to 1600 μg/ml)
   25 μl human rIL-2 (80 U/ml)
   25 μl mouse rIFNγ (4000 U/ml)
6. Pool lymph node cells (from Step 4), wash once in complete DMEM medium at 4°C and dilute them in complete DMEM medium at 1×10^3 cells/ml. Add 50 μl of these cells into each well of the plate prepared in Step 5 and incubate 7 days in a humidified 37°C, 5% CO_2 incubator.
7. Aspirate 50 μl of media and add 25 μl human rIL-2 (80 U/ml) and 25 μl mouse rIFNγ (4000 U/ml) to each well. Incubate for additional 5 to 7 days in a humidified 37°C, 5% CO_2 incubator.
8. Check under the microscope. Use only the wells with a single cluster of growing T cells.

Comments

1. One can use 100 μl of 50% MLC-supernatant instead of rIL-2 and rIFNγ.
2. This protocol results in production of Th1 cells. To prepare Th2 cells, add 50 μl of human rIL-2 (40 U/ml) or 50 μl 40% ConA-supernatant (instead of rIFNγ) at Steps 4 and 6.

B. *Maintaining Th clones*

Protocol

1. Add the following into a 24-well flat-bottom tissue culture plate:
   5×10^4 to 2×10^5 cloned T cells in 100 μl complete DMEM medium
   6×10^6 irradiated syngeneic spleen cells in 0.9 ml complete DMEM medium
   50 to 500 μg/ml of antigen
   For Th1 clones: human rIL-2 (25 U/ml) and mouse rIFNγ (250 U/ml) or 33% MLC-supernatant
   For Th2 clones: human rIL-2 (25 U/ml) or 10% ConA-supernatant
2. Cultivate cells in a humidified 37°C, 5% CO_2 incubator and subculture them every 7 days.

Comments

1. The concentrations of growth factors are final concentrations. For long-term cultivation, use 10 U/ml of IL-2.

1. ConA-supernatant

Materials and reagents

- Mouse spleen cells
- Complete DMEM medium with 5% FCS
- FCS
- 50-ml conical centrifuge tubes
- 25-cm² tissue culture flasks
- Concanavalin A (ConA; Sigma)
- Humidified 37°C, 5% CO_2 incubator

Protocol

1. Cultivate 1.25×10^6 spleen cells/ml for 24 to 48 hr with 2.5 μg/ml ConA in DMEM [without 3-(N-Morpholino)propanesulforic acid (MOPS)] containing 5% FCS in a humidified 37°C, 5% CO_2 incubator.

2. Collect culture supernatant and centrifuge at 800 × *g* for 10 min at 4°C.
3. Test ConA-supernatant for IL-2 content (see Chapter 6).

Comments

1. Rat spleen cells can be used instead of murine cells.

2. MLC-supernatant

Materials and reagents

- C57Bl/6 and DBA/2 mice
- DMEM medium with 5% FCS
- FCS
- 50-ml conical centrifuge tubes
- 25-cm² tissue culture flasks
- Humidified 37°C, 5% CO_2 incubator

Protocol

1. Mix 2.5 × 10^7 C57Bl/6 mouse spleen cells with the same number of irradiated (2000 to 4000 rad) DBA/2 mouse spleen cells in 20 ml complete DMEM medium with 5% FCS and incubate in upright 25-cm² plastic tissue culture flasks for 14 days in a humidified 37°C, 5% CO_2 incubator.
2. Collect cells in a 50-ml centrifuge tube and centrifuge at 200*g* at room temperature for 10 min. Discard supernatant and wash cells once with complete DMEM medium.
3. Mix 6 × 10^6 cells from Step 2 with 2.5 × 10^7 irradiated DBA/2 spleen cells in 20 ml complete DMEM medium with 5% FCS and incubate in an upright 50-ml plastic tissue culture flask for 36 hr in a humidified 37°C, 5% CO_2 incubator.
4. Collect culture supernatant and centrifuge at 800*g* for 10 min at 4°C.
5. Test MLC-supernatant for IL-2 and IFNγ content (see Chapter 6).

II. Preparation of human T cell clones

Both protocols for the generation of antigen-specific human T cell clones are based on use of mononuclear cells from an antigen-sensitized donor. The existence of natural and/or polyspecific antibodies (for review, see Reference 3) makes it possible to generate a human T cell clone even without immunization, but generally the chances are extremely low. The use of antigen-specific bulk cultures overcomes this problem; however, one must keep in mind that these cell populations are not clonal.

A. *Using stimulation/starving cycles*

Materials and reagents

- Peripheral blood mononuclear cells (see Chapter 1)
- Antigen
- RPMI 1640 medium with antibiotics, 25 m*M* HEPES
- RPMI 1640 medium with antibiotics, 25 m*M* HEPES, and 10% human AB serum
- Irradiated (3500 rad) autologous mononuclear cells (from the same donor)
- Human rIL-2
- Ficoll-Hypaque™
- 24-well, flat-bottom tissue culture plates
- 96-well, flat-bottom tissue culture plates
- Humidified 37°C, 5% CO_2 incubator

Protocol

1. Dilute mononuclear cells in RPMI 1640 medium containing 10% human AB serum to 2×10^6 cells/ml and add 2 ml of this suspension into wells of a 24-well plate.
2. Add optimal amount of antigen (5 to 500 μg/ml) and incubate 7 days in a humidified 37°C, 5% CO_2 incubator.
3. Pool all cells and wash once by centrifugation at $450 \times g$ in RPMI 1640 medium at room temperature. Discard supernatant and centrifuge cells through Ficoll-Hypaque gradient (see Chapter 1).
4. Recover cells, wash them 2× by centrifugation at 450*g* in RPMI 1640 medium at room temperature, and count them. Dilute the cells to 10^6 cells/ml in RPMI 1640 medium containing 10% human AB serum.
5. Add 1 ml of this cell suspension into each well of a 24-well plate. Add 1 ml of 3×10^6/ml of irradiated mononuclear cells into each well. Incubate 7 days in a humidified 37°C, 5% CO_2 incubator. *This is a starving cycle.*
6. Repeat Steps 3, 4, and 5 with the only exception of adding the optimal concentration of antigen in Step 5. *This is a stimulation cycle.*
7. Repeat starving and stimulation cycles 3× each.
8. Centrifuge cells through Ficoll-Hypaque gradient, wash 2× by centrifugation at 450*g* in RPMI 1640 medium at room temperature, and evaluate the antigen specificity by an antigen-specific proliferation assay (see Chapter 3).
9. Prepare clones by limiting dilution in 96-well plates containing:
   105 irradiated autologous mononuclear cells (per well)
   30 U/ml IL-2
   Antigen
   T cells from Step 8 (plate 0.3, 1, and 3 cells per well)

10. Incubate 7 days in a humidified 37°C, 5% CO_2 incubator. Check under the microscope. Use only those wells with a single cluster of growing T cells.
11. Transfer single clusters of growing cells to 24-well plates with irradiated autologous mononuclear cells and antigen and incubate for 7 days in a humidified 37°C, 5% CO_2 incubator.
12. Check the growing cells for antigen specificity (see Chapter 3).
13. Continue cultivation and expansion of antigen-specific clones by repeating starving and stimulation cycles.

Comments

1. The optimal antigen concentration should be determined before the experiment, either by a test of lymphokine production (see Chapter 6) or T cell proliferation (see Chapter 3).
2. The optimal dose for irradiation of mononuclear cells should be determined in a preliminary experiment.

B. *Antigen-nonspecific T cell clones*[4]

Materials and reagents

- Peripheral blood mononuclear cells (see Chapter 1)
- RPMI 1640 medium with antibiotics, 25 m*M* HEPES, and 10% human AB serum
- Irradiated (3500 rad) autologous mononuclear cells (from the same donor)
- Irradiated (3500 rad) allogeneic mononuclear cells (from a different donor)
- Human rIL-2
- Phytohemagglutinin (PHA)
- Ficoll-Hypaque™
- 24-well, flat-bottom tissue culture plates
- 96-well, flat-bottom tissue culture plates
- Humidified 37°C, 5% CO_2 incubator

Protocol

1. Isolate T lymphocytes from peripheral blood mononuclear cells (see Chapter 1).
2. Using a 24-well, flat-bottom tissue culture plate, mix into each well 10^5 T cells with 5×10^4 irradiated autologous cells in a final volume of 2 ml complete RPMI medium containing 5 μg/ml PHA. Incubate for 4 days in a humidified 37°C, 5% CO_2 incubator.

3. Aspirate 1 ml supernatant and add 1 ml fresh medium supplemented with 50 U rIL-2. Incubate for 3 days in a humidified 37°C, 5% CO_2 incubator.
4. Centrifuge cells through a Ficoll-Hypaque™ gradient, wash twice by centrifugation at 450*g* in RPMI 1640 medium at room temperature, and count them.
5. Put 105 irradiated allogeneic cells, 5 μg/ml PHA, and 25 U/ml rIL-2 (final volume of 200 μl) into each well of a 96-well, flat-bottom tissue culture plate. Plate T cells (from Step 4) into each well (plate 0.3, 1, and 3 cells per well). Incubate for several days in a humidified 37°C, 5% CO_2 incubator.
6. Aspirate 100 μl supernatant and add 100 μl complete medium supplemented with 50 U/ml rIL-2. Incubate for an additional 3 to 4 days in a humidified 37°C, 5% CO_2 incubator.
7. Aspirate 100 μl supernatant and add 5×10^4 irradiated allogeneic cells, 5 mg/ml PHA and 50 U/ml rIL-2 (final volume 200 μl). Incubate for additional 4 days in a humidified 37°C, 5% CO_2 incubator.
8. Repeat Step 6. At the end of incubation, identify wells with growing clones under a microscope and expand growing cultures by repeating Steps 6 and 7.

C. *Long-term maintenance of antigen-specific and nonspecific T cell clones*

Materials and reagents

- Ficoll-Hypaque
- T cell clones
- RPMI 1640 medium with antibiotics, 25 m*M* HEPES
- RPMI 1640 medium with antibiotics, 25 m*M* HEPES with 10% human AB serum
- Human rIL-2
- PHA
- 24-well, flat-bottom tissue culture plates
- Irradiated (3500 rad) allogeneic mononuclear cells (from a different donor)
- Humidified 37°C, 5% CO_2 incubator

Protocol

1. Centrifuge cells through a Ficoll-Hypaque gradient, wash 2× by centrifugation at 450*g* in serum-free RPMI 1640 medium at room temperature, count them, and resuspend at 10^6 cells/ml in complete RPMI 1640 medium.
2. Plate 1 ml of this suspension into each well of a 24-well plate.

3. Add 1 ml irradiated allogeneic mononuclear cells (2×10^6 cells/ml) with 5 μg/ml PHA and 15 U/ml rIL-2 into each well. Incubate the plate for 4 days in a humidified 37°C, 5% CO_2 incubator.
4. Aspirate 1 ml supernatant and add 1 ml fresh complete RPMI 1640 medium supplemented with 25 U/ml rIL-2. Incubate for an additional 3 days in a humidified 37°C, 5% CO_2 incubator.
5. Pool the growing T cells. Centrifuge pooled cells through Ficoll-Hypaque™ gradient, wash 2× by centrifugation at 450*g* in serum-free RPMI 1640 medium at room temperature, count them, and resuspend at 10^6 cells/ml in complete RPMI 1640 medium.
6. Repeat Steps 3, 4, and 5 every week.

Comments

1. The above-described protocol is for antigen-nonspecific T cell clones. To maintain antigen-specific T cell clones, stimulate them once a month with irradiated autologous mononuclear cells and antigen. Incubate the mixture of T cells and irradiated cells (at a ratio of 1:3) with the antigen for 7 days in a humidified 37°C, 5% CO_2 incubator.

D. *Bulk cultures of antigen-specific T helper cells*[5]

Materials and reagents

- Peripheral blood mononuclear cells
- Human rIL-2
- AIM V medium (Gibco)
- AIM V medium supplemented with 2.5% autologous serum
- Antigen
- Ficoll-Hypaque
- 75-cm^2 tissue culture flasks
- Humidified 37°C, 5% CO_2 incubator

Protocol

1. Incubate 2×10^7 peripheral blood mononuclear cells in serum-free AIM V medium supplemented with 30 μg/ml of antigen (total volume of 25 ml/flask) for 3 days in a humidified 37°C, 5% CO_2 incubator.
2. Pool nonadherent cells, isolated by washing the culture flasks 3× with AIM V medium, and wash them once by centrifugation in AIM V medium for 10 min at 450*g* at room temperature.

3. Incubate these cells for an additional 14 days in AIM V medium with 2.5% autologous serum, 30 µg/ml of antigen and 30 U/ml rIL-2 (total volume of 25 ml/flask) in a humidified 37°C, 5% CO_2 incubator.
4. Centrifuge cells through Ficoll-Hypaque™ gradient, wash 2× by centrifugation at 450*g* in desired medium at room temperature, count them, and resuspend for further experiments.

E. Preparation of T cell hybridomas[6]

T cell hybridomas were first introduced in 1987 by Kontiainen et al.[7] They are usually prepared by fusing tumor cells with activated T lymphocytes. The resulting heterogeneous population can be subsequently cloned. The advantage of this technique is the fact that obtained hybridomas can be easily grown in large numbers in the absence of expensive growth factors. The basic principles are identical to those of B cell hybridomas (Chapter 8); that is, they do not require components other than those of normal medium and serum. One of the disadvantages is the lower genetical stability compared to normal cells, this being due to frequent chromosome shedding. In addition, the most common tumor parent of the T cell hybridomas is a mouse thymoma BW5147. Cells derived from this line have changed expression of CD4 and CD8 markers. Despite these potential setbacks, T cell hybridomas have been used in researching almost all aspects of T cell biology. Readers seeking additional information should refer to References 8 through 13.

Materials and reagents

- BW5147 cell line (ATCC TIB 48)
- Dulbecco's medium supplemented with 10% FCS, 2×10^{-5} *M* mercaptoethanol, and antibiotics
- HAT (Sigma): 1 ml of 50× concentrated powder (diluted in 10 ml medium without FCS) per 50 ml medium
- HT (Sigma): 1 ml of 50× concentrated powder (diluted in 10 ml medium without FCS) per 50 ml medium
- Dulbecco's medium without any supplements
- Freshly isolated primed T cells (see Chapter 1; see below)
- Polyethylene glycol (PEG; Sigma), 50% w/w in Dulbecco's medium without any supplements
- 50-ml conical polypropylene centrifuge tubes
- 96-well tissue culture plates
- 1-ml pipettes
- 10-ml pipettes
- Glass beakers
- Humidified 5% CO_2 incubators

Protocol

(*Note*: All reagents and materials must be sterile. Use appropriate sterile techniques throughout the procedure.)

1. Split BW5147 cells before fusion and harvest while they are still in log phase (see *Comments*).
2. Store conditioned medium.
3. Wash BW5147 cells 3× with serum-free Dulbecco's medium by centrifugation at 500*g* for 5 min at room temperature.
4. In a 50-ml tube, mix 10^7 BW 5147 cells with 5×10^7 T cells, add 30 ml serum-free Dulbecco's medium and spin by centrifugation at 500*g* for 5 min at room temperature.
5. Pour off supernatant.
6. Disperse the pellet and add 1 ml prewarmed 50% PEG.
7. Gently resuspend the pellet by a single passage through a 10-ml pipette.
8. Incubate at 37°C for 45 sec.
9. Spin by centrifugation at 500*g* for 5 min at room temperature.
10. Pour off supernatant.
11. Wash down the pellet with Dulbecco's medium (with FCS and 2-ME) without resuspension of the pellet.
12. Add 10 ml Dulbecco's medium (with FCS and 2-ME) and resuspend by several passages through a 10-ml pipette.
13. Add an additional 40 ml Dulbecco's medium (with FCS and 2-ME) to the cell suspension.
14. Aliquot at 0.1 ml/well into four 96-well tissue culture plates.
15. Repeat Steps 13 and 14 twice.
16. Cultivate the plates at 37°C in a humidified, 5 % CO_2 incubator.
17. Three days after the fusion, add 0.05 ml Dulbecco's medium (with FCS and 2-ME) containing 3× concentration of HAT into each well.
18. Change the medium completely every 5 days.
19. After day 7, start screening the wells for hybridoma growth. Transfer the good clusters into wells of 24-well tissue culture plates and add 1.5 ml Dulbecco's medium (with FCS and 2-ME) with HAT into each well.
20. After day 15, change medium in all wells with growing hybridomas into Dulbecco's medium (with FCS and 2-ME) with HT.
21. Screen positive wells, depending on the purpose of the fusion, clone the desirable T cell hybridomas, and freeze them.

Comments

1. Log phase ends approximately when cell density is around 7×10^5 cells/ml.
2. Store conditioned medium several days before the actual fusion.

3. Steps 13 and 14 are repeated 2× due to difficulties in predicting how many hybridomas will eventually appear.

1. In vivo *priming of T cells*[6]

Priming of T cells prior fusion corresponds to immunization of B lymphocytes prior production of B cell hybridomas. Each laboratory involved in T cell hybridomas has a preferred method for priming.

Materials and reagents

- Antigen
- Complete Freund's adjuvant (Sigma)
- Mice
- Cutting board
- 60 × 15-mm Petri dishes
- Dulbecco's medium (with FCS and 2-ME; see above)
- 15-ml conical centrifuge tubes
- Click's medium supplemented with 1% fresh mouse serum, 863 μg/ml sodium bicarbonate, 5×10^{-5} *M* 2-mercaptoethanol and antibiotics
- Ficoll-Hypaque™
- 24-well tissue culture plates
- BSS containing 15% FCS
- Human recombinant IL-2
- 25-cm^2 tissue culture flasks
- Humidified 10% CO_2 incubators

Protocol

1. Prepare the antigen by emulsification in complete Freund's adjuvant as described in Chapter 8.
2. Immunize the mice according to the standard laboratory protocols, either into the base of the tail or subcutaneously.
3. Harvest the lymph nodes and prepare cell suspension according to the protocol described in Chapter 1.
4. Resuspend lymph node cells at 4×10^6 cells/ml in Click's medium.
5. Add 1.5 ml cell suspension into wells of the 24-well tissue culture plates and incubate for 4 days at 37°C in humidified 10% CO_2 incubator.
6. Harvest the cells and wash by centrifugation at 1000*g* for 10 min at 4°C.
7. Resuspend in 5 ml BSS supplemented with 15% FCS.
8. Put 2 ml Ficoll-Hypaque into a 15-ml conical tube, carefully add 5 ml cell suspension on top of the Ficoll-Hypaque and spin at 1500*g* for 15 min at room temperature.
9. Harvest the living cells from the interface between Ficoll and BSS.

10. Wash once by centrifugation at 300*g* for 5 min at 4°C.
11. Resuspend at 1 × 10^5 cells/ml in complete Dulbecco's medium (with FCS and 2-ME) containing 3 IU/ml rIL-2.
12. Incubate in 25-cm^2 tissue culture flasks in a humidified 10% CO_2 incubator for 3 days.
13. Harvest, wash by centrifugation, and measure the viability.

Comments

1. Lymph nodes are harvested according to the sites of injection. In mice, immunization in the base of the tail is considered to be the best, and the adequate lymph nodes are the periaortic and inguinals. Large animals such as rats or hamsters are immunized subcutaneously and the draining lymph nodes are branchial and axillary.
2. In case of a high percentage of dead cells after Step 13, dead cells might again be removed using another Ficoll-Hypaque™ gradient (Step 8).

III. Preparation of human B cell clone[14]

Materials and reagents

- Marmoset B95-8 cell line releasing EVB (CRL-1612; ATCC)
- RPMI 1640 medium with 10% FCS
- Cyclosporin A (Sandoz)
- 96-well, flat-bottom tissue culture plates (Costar)
- 25-cm^2 tissue culture flasks (Costar)
- Ethanol
- Human rIL-2
- 15-ml conical centrifuge tubes
- 0.22-μm filter (Costar)
- Humidified 37°C, 5% CO_2 incubator

Protocol

1. Incubate the B95-8 cell line in tissue culture flasks in RPMI 1640 medium containing 10% FCS. Collect the cell-free supernatant and filter it by passing through the 0.22-μm filter.
2. Isolate mononuclear cells from peripheral blood (see Chapter 1). Resuspend 10^7 of washed (at least 5×; centrifugation at 300*g* for 5 min at 4°C) mononuclear cells in 10 ml RPMI 1640 with 10% FCS, and 30% supernatant of the B95-8 cell line and 600 ng/ml cyclosporin A (dissolve in ethanol at 1 mg/ml).
3. Incubate for 16 hr at 37°C. Wash the cells 3× in RPMI 1640 medium with 10% FCS at 250*g* for 10 min.

4. Cultivate cells at concentration 5×10^4 cells/well in 96-well, flat-bottom tissue culture plates in 200 μl RPMI 1640 with 10% FCS and 600 ng/ml cyclosporin A for 13 days.
5. Clone cells by limiting dilution.

Comments

1. The optimal time for initial incubation with EBV-containg B95-8-derived supernatant may vary.

IV. Cloning by limiting dilution technique

In the process of selecting hybridomas, T cell or B cell lines of the desired specificity, a final but very important step is the selection of a clonal cell population. This will ensure not only that the antibodies and/or cell lines have a single specificity, but will help prevent the overgrowth of variants that have lost the desired phenotype. In the case of hybridoma selection, for example, positive wells may contain cells derived from more than one clone; or even if derived from a single hybridoma, chromosome loss may result in the appearance of a nonsecreting progeny of cells that might overgrow antibody-secreting cells. In addition, subcloning may also allow the selection of high-antibody secreting variants.

Several techniques have been used for cloning purposes, including the following.

1. *Cloning in soft agar.* In this technique, cells are diluted and cultured in soft-agar plates[15] so that cell clones will grow as colonies (arising from a single cell precursor) at different locations on the plate. Because the agar prevents the cells from moving and mixing, the clonality of the colonies is ensured. This technique, however, presents some disadvantages, including:
   a. The cloning efficiency may be relatively low compared to other techniques, such as limiting dilution.
   b. The cells grown as colonies need to be adapted to liquid culture.
   c. In the case of hybridomas, the cells need to be grown as liquid cultures and supernatants generated before they can be screened.
2. *Limiting dilution.* In this technique, the cells are first diluted and cultured in 96- or 24-well tissue culture plates at cell densities at which, statistically (Poisson distribution), most of the wells would contain only a single cell. Many variations of this basic technique exist, depending on the nature of the cells being cloned and their need for stimulation and/or growth factors. For example, several limiting dilution techniques for the cloning of hybridomas differ in their use of "feeder" cells or "conditioned supernatants" from thymocytes, splenic cells, or growth factor-producing cell lines (e.g.,

P388D_1 cells and IL-6).[16] On the other hand, cloning of antigen-specific T cells might require the presence of antigen-presenting cells, antigen, and IL-2.

3. *Cloning by micromanipulation*. Repeated micromanipulation[17] is recommended as the only method that really ensures clonality. Otherwise, it is not possible to ascertain that any clone obtained by either limiting dilution or soft agar culture has in reality been produced by a single T cell.
4. *Other techniques*. Cloning of positive hybridomas has also been done using the fluorescence-activated cell sorter (FACS).[18] In this technique, the FACS can be used to first select positive hybridomas based on the binding of a fluorescent antigen, while at the same time sorting the positive cells onto 96-well tissue culture plates at 1 cell per well.

Because of its simplicity and lack of dependence on sophisticated equipment, only the limiting dilution technique is further discussed in this chapter. The method described is used for the limiting dilution cloning of hybridomas. Whereas the basic technique is the same, cloning of T cell lines requires different conditions, particularly antigen and accessory cells.

Materials and reagents

- Candidate cells (primary hybridomas)
- Cloning medium: DMEM containing 20% heat-inactivated fetal calf serum (FCS), 4.5 g/l glucose, 100 U/ml penicillin, 100 μg/ml streptomycin, and 20% conditioned medium from SP2/0-Ag14 cells (ATCC Cat. No. CRL 1581)
- Culture medium: DMEM containing 10% heat-inactivated fetal calf serum (FCS), 4.5 g/l glucose, 100 U/ml penicillin, and 100 μg/ml streptomycin.
- 96-well tissue culture plates (flat bottom)
- 15- and 50-ml centrifuge tubes
- Multichannel pipette
- Sterile troughs
- Pasteur pipettes
- Inverted microscope
- Centrifuge (set at 4°C)
- Incubator (humidified, set at 37°C and 5% CO_2)
- Reagents and materials necessary for hybridoma screening

Protocol

(*Note*: All reagents and materials must be sterile. Use appropriate sterile techniques throughout the procedure.)

1. Resuspend the candidate hybridoma by pipetting gently with the aid of a sterile Pasteur pipette. Transfer the cells to a 15-ml centrifuge tube and assess viability by Trypan blue exclusion.
2. Readjust the cell density to 1×10^5 cells/ml using culture medium. Initially, prepare a 1:20 dilution of the cells in cloning medium by pipetting 0.1 ml of the original cell suspension and diluting it into 1.9 ml of medium. Next, prepare a 1:100 dilution by pipetting 0.25 ml of this suspension (1:20) and mixing it with 24.75 ml cloning medium (this suspension should now contain 50 cells/ml). Finally, prepare a 5 cells/ml suspension by diluting 2.0 ml of the 50 cells/ml suspension and mixing it with 18.0 ml cloning medium. The cloning medium must be prewarmed at 37°C.
3. Seed one 96-well tissue culture plate with 200 μl/well of the 50 cells/ml suspension and another plate with 200 μl/well of the 5 cells/ml suspension. On average, the two plates should contain 10 and 1 cells/well, respectively.
4. Incubate the plates in a humidified, 37°C, 5% CO_2 incubator for approximately 7 to 14 days. In the meantime, check the plates under an inverted microscope to ascertain growth and the presence of single or multiple colonies in each well. Eventually, colonies will become visible macroscopically.
5. If adequate growth (most wells contain single colonies only) is detected in the plate seeded at 1 cell/well, use this plate for screening and selection. If not, use the plate seeded at 10 cells/well, making sure that, if possible, only those wells exhibiting a single colony are used.
6. When the colony covers approximately 10 to 20% of the surface of the well, remove 100 μl supernatant and test for the desired specificity. Feed the wells with 100 μl fresh cloning medium. Feed the cells at any time if the medium becomes acidic (yellow) by aspirating approximately 100 μl supernatant and replacing it with 100 μl fresh cloning medium.
7. Select the desired hybridomas based on the screening. Expand to a 24-well plate. Feed the cells every 2 to 3 days by removing half of the supernatant and replacing it with medium. At this point, the cells can be gradually adapted to growth in culture medium (10% FCS) without the conditioned medium by substituting culture medium for the cloning medium in the feeding schedule.
8. If questions remain about the clonality of the hybridomas selected, repeat the procedure (Steps 1 to 7) one more time.

Comments

1. The choice of a high-quality fetal calf serum of proven hybridoma-supporting capacity (e.g., Hyclone, Sigma) is essential.

2. For preparation of conditioned medium from SP2/0-Ag14 cells, seed cells in a 75-cm^2 culture flask at a initial cell density of 1×10^5 cells/ml, using culture medium (DMEM-10% FCS). The SP2/0-Ag14 should be routinely screened for mycoplasma contamination. Use only cells that have been proven mycoplasma-free.
3. The reason for plating cells at 10 and 1 cells/well is that primary hybridomas will usually exhibit less than 100% plating efficiency.
4. Aliquots of cells must be frozen whenever sufficient numbers can be obtained (Step 7).

References

1. Fitch, F.W. and Gajewski, T.F., Production of T cell clones, in *Current Protocols in Immunology,* Coligan, J.E., Kruisbeek, A.M., Margulies, D.H., Shevach, E.M., and Strober, W., Eds., Greene Publishing and Wiley InterScience, New York, 1991, 3.13.1.
2. Gajewski, T.F., Joyce, J., and Fitch, F.W., Anti-proliferative effect on IFN-gamma in immune regulation. III. Differential selection of T_h1 and T_h2 murine helper T lymphocyte clones using rIL-2 and rIFN-gamma, *J. Immunol.,* 143, 15, 1989.
3. Shoenfeld, Y. and Isenberg, D.A., Eds., *Natural Antibodies. Their Physiological Role and Regulatory Significance,* CRC Press, Boca Raton, FL, 1993.
4. Nutman, T.B., Long-term and immortalized human cell lines and clones, in *Current Protocols in Immunology,* Coligan, J.E., Kruisbeek, A.M., Margulies, D.H., Shevach, E.M., and Strober, W., Eds., Greene Publ. and Wiley Inter-Science, New York, 1992, 7.19.1.
5. Gosselin, E.J., Wardwell, K., Gosselin, D.R., Alter, N., Fisher, J.L., and Guyre, P.M., Enhanced antigen presentation using human Fcγ receptor (monocyte/macrophage)-specific immunogens, *J. Immunol.,* 149, 3477, 1992.
6. White, J., Kappler, J., and Marrack, P., Production and characterization of T cell hybridomas, *Meth. Mol. Biol.,* 134, 185, 2000.
7. Kontiainen, S., Simpson, E., Bohler, E., Beverly, P.C.L., Herzenberg, L.A., Firzpatrick, W.A., Vogt, P., Torano, A., McKenzie, I.F.C., and Feldman, M., T cell line producing antigen-specific suppressor factor, *Nature,* 274, 477, 1987.
8. Waters, S.J., Winchester, R.J., Nagase, F., Thorbecke, G.J., and Bona, C.A., Antigen presentation by murine and human cells to a murine T-cell hybridoma: demonstration of a restriction element associated with a major histocompatibility complex class II determinant(s) shared by both species, *Proc. Natl. Acad. Sci. U.S.A.,* 81, 7559, 1984.
9. Boen, E., Crownover, A.R., McIlhaney, M., Korman, A.J., and Bill, J., Identification of T cell ligands in a library of peptides covalently attached to HLA-DR4, *J. Immunol.,* 165, 2040, 2000.
10. Kovalik, J.P., Singh, N., Mendiratta, S.K., Martin, W.D., Ignatowicz, L., and Van Kaer, L., The alloreactive and self-restricted $CD4^+$ T cell response directed against a single MHC class II/peptide combination, *J. Immunol.,* 165, 1285, 2000.
11. Viret, C., Lantz, O., He, X., Bendelac, A., and Janeway, C.A., A NK1.1 thymocyte-derived TCR β-chain transgene promotes positive selection of thymic α/β T cells, *J. Immunol.,* 165, 3004, 2000.

12. Popovic, P., Colic, M., Vucevic, D., Gasic, S., and Pavicic, L., Comparison of signaling pathways involved in apoptosis of a thymocyte hybridoma triggered by a rat thymic medullary epithelial cell line, dexamethasone or T-cell receptor cross-linking, *Immunology Lett.*, 72, 83, 2000.
13. McInerney, M.F., Burkey, J., Guan, L., Flynn, J.C., Oravecz, K.I., and Janeway, C.A., An islet-specific $CD8^+$ T cell hybridoma generated from non-obese diabetic mice recognizes insulin as an autoantigen, *Diabetes Res. Clin. Practice*, 47, 151, 2000.
14. Lanzavecchia, A., Antigen-specific interaction between T and B cells, *Nature*, 314, 537, 1985.
15. Goding, J.W., Antibody production by hybridomas, *J. Immunol. Methods*, 39, 285, 1980.
16. Yokoyama, W.M., Production of monoclonal antibodies, in *Current Protocols in Immunology*, Coligan, J.E., Kruisbeek, A.M., Margulies, D.H., Shevach, E.M., and Strober, W., Eds., Greene Publ. and Wiley InterScience, New York, 1992, 2.5.1.
17. Glasenbook, A.L. and Fitch, F.W., Derivation of T cell clones, in *Monoclonal Antibodies and Functional Cell Lines*, Kenneth, R.H., Bechtol, K.B., and McKearn, T.J., Eds., Plenum Press, New York, 1984, 413.
18. Parks, D.R., Bryan, V.M., Oi, V.T., and Herzenberg, L.A., Antigen-specific identification and cloning of hybridomas with a fluorescence-activated cell sorter, *Proc. Natl. Acad. Sci. U.S.A.*, 76, 1962–1966, 1979.

chapter five

Cytotoxic cells

Contents

I. Cell-mediated cytotoxicity

Cell mediated cytotoxicity is a general term including three different mechanisms: antibody-dependent cell-mediated cytotoxicity (ADCC), natural killer (NK)/lymphokine-activated killer (LAK) cell cytotoxicity, and T cell cytotoxicity. In an ADCC cytotoxic reaction, effector cells mediate target cell lysis by binding their Fc receptors to the Fc fragment of antibodies bound to target cells. The other two mechanisms occur without a need for antibodies.

Several different ways of target cell labeling for the assessment of cytotoxic activity have been used. The two most common techniques use ^{51}Cr release[1-3] from ^{51}Cr-labeled targets or an enzymatic assay measuring release of intracellular substances. All these methods are based on measuring cell death judged from plasma membrane disintegration and the consequent release of cytoplasm. DNA fragmentation, a common event occurring during apoptosis, is also an early event in the cell death caused by cytotoxic cells.[4] The JAM test[5] is a sensitive and easy test for DNA fragmentation and cell death.

A. *ADCC*[6]

Materials and reagents

- RPMI-1640 medium with 25m*M* HEPES and 10% FCS
- 5% (v/v) Triton X-100 (Sigma)
- 6-ml plastic centrifuge tubes
- 96-well, round-bottom microtiter plates with cover (Costar)
- 15-ml conical centrifuge tubes
- Tubes suitable for your γ-counter
- γ-counter
- 75-cm² tissue culture flask (Costar)
- ^{51}Cr-labeled target cells (see Section D)
- Ficoll-Hypaque™-separated peripheral blood cells (see Chapter 1) or purified NK cells
- Humidified 37°C, 5% CO_2 incubator

Protocol

1. Dilute effector cells to 1×10^7/ml in medium and antibody-coated and non-antibody-coated ^{51}CR-labeled target cells to 1×10^5/ml in medium.
2. Prepare 0.8 ml each of 1:2, 1:4, and 1:8 dilutions of effector cells in medium using 6-ml centrifuge tubes.
3. Pipettete 0.1 ml undiluted effector cells from left to right along a row of a 96-well, round-bottom microtiter plate for each assay condition. Make a duplicate row in the same fashion. Repeat for the 1:2, 1:4, and 1:8 dilutions. Leave one row empty for each condition.
4. Add 0.1 ml antibody-coated ^{51}Cr-labeled target cells to the first row and 0.1 ml non-antibody-coated ^{51}Cr-labeled target cells to the second row for each condition. Add 0.1 ml antibody-coated ^{51}Cr-labeled target cells into the first six wells of an empty row, and 0.1 ml non-antibody-coated ^{51}Cr-labeled target cells into the other six wells.
5. Add 0.1 ml of 5% Triton X-100 to three of the wells containing antibody-coated target cells and non-antibody-coated target cells. Add 0.1 ml medium into remaining control wells.
6. Centrifuge the plates for 3 min at 100*g* at room temperature.
7. Incubate for 18 hr in a humidified 37°C, 5% CO_2 incubator.
8. Centrifuge the plates for 5 min at 550*g* at room temperature. Carefully transfer the supernatants into small tubes optimal for your γ-counter.

B. *CytoTox 96™ cytotoxicity assay*

This method is a colorimetric nonradioactive alternative to the traditional ^{51}Cr-release-based cytotoxicity techniques. The assay measures lactate dehydrogenase release from lysed cells. Besides easier handling, mostly because of it being nonradioactive, another advantage of this technique is its much longer expiration time compared to the rather short half-life of ^{51}Cr (27.7 days). Therefore, it is particularly useful to employ CytoTox 96™ when performing cytotoxicity experiments only occasionally. The sensitivity of this assay is fully comparable to the ^{51}Cr-release assay[7-8]; however, this technique cannot be used for evaluation of erythrocyte lysis.

Materials and reagents

- Isolated NK cells
- Target cells
- RPMI 1640 medium
- CytoTox 96™ cytotoxicity assay (Promega)
- V- or round-bottom 96-well plates (Costar)
- ELISA reader equipped with 490-nm filter

Protocol

1. Add target and effector cells to wells according to experimental protocol.
2. Add cells for spontaneous release control, maximum release control, and effector cell release control.
3. Add culture medium and lysis solution for volume correction control.
4. Add culture medium for culture medium background.
5. Centrifuge plates at 250*g* for 4 min at room temperature.
6. Incubate plates for 4 hr at 37°C.
7. Add lysis solution (10 µl per 100 µl of supernatant) 45 min prior to further centrifugation.
8. Centrifuge plates at 250*g* for 4 min at room temperature.
9. Transfer 50 µl of supernatant from each well into a new, round-bottom, 96-well plate.
10. Add 50 µl reconstituted substrate mix (12 ml assay buffer added to a bottle of substrate mix; once resuspended, protect from light and store at –20°C for up to 2 months) to each well with the transferred supernatant.
11. Incubate plates for 30 min at room temperature.
12. Add 50 µl of stop solution and read absorbance at 490 nm.

Comments

1. Volume correction control adjusts for the volume changes caused by addition of the lysis solution. Culture medium background corrects for LDH activity caused by the level of animal sera and by the presence of phenol red in medium. One can skip this step by using a phenol red-free medium and by lowering the amount of serum.

2. As the content of lactate dehydrogenase in various target cells varies, preliminary experiments for optimization of their number are recommended.

C. *LAK/NK cytotoxicity*

Materials and reagents

- Effector cells
- RPMI 1640 medium with 25 m*M* HEPES and 10% FCS
- 5% (v/v) Triton X-100
- 6-ml plastic centrifuge tubes
- 96-well, round-bottom microtiter plates with cover (Costar)
- 15-ml conical centrifuge tubes
- Tubes suitable for your γ-counter
- γ-counter
- ^{51}Cr-labeled target cells (see Section D)
- 2% SDS
- Ficoll-Hypaque-separated peripheral blood cells (see Chapter 1) or purified NK cells
- Humidified 37°C, 5% CO_2 incubator

Protocol

1. Dilute effector cells to appropriate concentration, depending on the experimental design. It is recommended that one use three different effector:target ratios. The actual ratio used is dependent on factors such as target sensitivity and the effector cell potency.
2. Add 100 μl of effector cells into wells of the 96-well round-bottom microtiter plates in triplicate. Leave row A blank.
3. Add 100 μl of medium into the first three wells of row A for spontaneous ^{51}Cr release control.
4. Add 50 μl of ^{51}Cr-labeled target cells to each well containing effector cells and to the second three wells of row A. These three wells will serve as a maximum lysis control.
5. Cover the plate and centrifuge it at 50*g* for 5 min at room temperature with brake off.
6. Incubate the plate for 4 hr in a humidified 37°C, 5% CO_2 incubator.
7. Add 100 μl of 2% SDS into those wells for maximum lysis control (second three wells, row A).
8. Transfer 50 μl of supernatant into the counting tubes and measure the radioactivity of the samples in a γ-counter.
9. Calculation.

$$\% \text{ Lysis} = \frac{\text{Experimental cpm} - \text{Spontaneous cpm}}{\text{Maximum cpm} - \text{Spontaneous cpm}} \times 100$$

D. ^{51}Cr-labeling

Materials and reagents

- Target cells
- $Na_2{}^{51}CrO_4$, 5 mCi/ml, specific activity 250 to 500 mCi/mg (Amersham)
- RPMI 1640 medium with 25 m*M* HEPES and 10% FCS
- 15-ml conical centrifuge tubes
- Tubes suitable for your γ-counter
- γ-counter

Protocol

1. Resuspend cells in medium at a concentration 1×10^7/ml. Check the viability; use only cells with viability higher than 95%.
2. Add $Na_2{}^{51}CrO_4$ to the cells (500 μCi per 1×10^7 cells) and incubate for 60 min at 37°C with occasional shaking.
3. Wash the cells at least 5× by centrifugation at 3000*g* for 10 min at room temperature. Check the radioactivity in the supernatant from the previous centrifugation. If still significantly higher than a background, repeat the washing procedure.

Comments

1. A major disadvantage of this very common technique is the rather high spontaneous ^{51}Cr release from target cells, especially when the cells are grown in monolayers and need to be trypsinized to obtain a single cell suspension prior to labeling.

E. Isolation of NK cells

Materials and reagents

- Blood
- 15-ml conical centrifuge tubes
- RPMI 1640 medium with 10% FCS
- Materials for isolation of mononuclear cells, panning, nylon wool column, and Percoll separation (see Chapter 1)
- 15-ml glass centrifuge tubes

Protocol

1. Isolate mononuclear cells from peripheral blood (see Chapter 1).
2. After five washes in medium (250*g* for 5 min at 4°C), deplete the suspension of monocytes and some B cells by panning (see Chapter 1).
3. After two washes in medium (250*g* for 5 min at 4°C), pass the cells through a nylon wool column to remove T cells.
4. After two additional washes in medium (250*g* for 5 min at 4°C), fractionate cells on a discontinuous Percoll gradient[9] (see Table 5.1).
5. Carefully layer 5 to 10 × 10^6 cells on top of the gradient and centrifuge at 550*g* for 30 min at room temperature with brakes off.
6. Collect cells from resulting bands and wash them twice with RPMI 1640 medium by centrifugation at 300*g* for 5 min at room temperature. NK cells are usually present in the first two bands from the top, between the low-density fractions.[9]

Table 5.1 Discontinuous Percoll Density Gradient

Fraction	Percoll[a] (ml)	Density (g/ml)	Volume[b] (ml)
1	2.55	1.053	2.5
2	2.70	1.060	2.5
3	2.85	1.063	2.5
4	3.00	1.068	1.5
5	3.15	1.073	1.5
6	3.30	1.077	1.5
7	4.00	1.080	1.5

[a] Stock solution.

[b] Volume of each fraction in a 15-ml glass centrifuge tube.

Comments

1. Individual steps can be substituted with the negative selection using magnetic microspheres coupled with appropriate antibodies (see Chapter 1). Another possibility is to use a positive selection using magnetic microspheres coupled with CD56 and CD16 antibodies.

F. *Generation of LAK cells*

Materials and reagents

- Isolated NK cells
- RPMI 1640 medium with 10% FCS

- Human rIL-2
- 25-cm^2 tissue culture flasks

Protocol

1. Resuspend isolated NK cells (1 × 10^6/ml) in RPMI 1640 medium containing 1000 U/ml rIL-2.
2. Put 10 ml of cell suspension into 25-cm^2 tissue culture flasks and incubate for 3 days in a humidified 37°C, 5% CO_2 incubator.
3. Shake the flasks well to remove all adherent cells. Rinse the flasks with RPMI 1640 medium. Centrifuge LAK cells twice in RPMI 1640 medium without rIL-2 at 500*g* for 5 min at room temperature. Count the cells.

G. *Proliferation of NK cells*[10]

Materials and reagents

- Isolated NK cells
- Peripheral blood mononuclear cells (see Chaper 1)
- RPMI 1640 medium with 2.5% human AB serum
- RPMI 1640 medium with 15% human AB serum
- Ionomycin (Calbiochem)
- 25-cm^2 and 150-cm^2 tissue culture flasks
- Daudi cells (ATCC; CCL-213)
- PMA (Sigma)
- PHA (Sigma)
- Humidified 37°C, 5% CO_2 incubator

Protocol

1. Prepare leukocyte conditioned medium (LCM): incubate 4 × 10^8 isolated peripheral blood mononuclear cells from each of two donors with 2.5 × 10^8 irradiated (8000 rad) Daudi cells in 500 ml RPMI 1640 medium with 2.5% human AB serum containing 10 ng/ml PMA and 4 μg/ml PHA in a 150-cm^2 tissue culture flasks for 120 min at 37°C. Wash the cells 3× in medium and resuspend in RPMI 1640 medium with 2.5% human AB serum. Incubate in the same flask for 48 hr at 37°C and collect the cell-free supernatant.
2. Incubate 1 × 10^6 purified NK cells/ml in 25-cm^2 tissue culture flasks in RPMI 1640 medium with 15% human AB serum, 20% LCM, and 750 ng/ml ionomycin for 24 hr in a humidified 37°C, 5% CO_2 incubator. Resuspend the cells in RPMI 1640 medium with 15% human AB serum and 20% LCM and incubate in the same flask for 10 to 14 days. Add fresh 20% LCM to keep concentration of 1 to 2 × 10^6 cells/ml.

Comments

1. LCM can be passed through a 0.45-μ filter and stored at –70°C.
2. It is important not to incubate cells in medium supplemented with ionomycin for more than 24 hr, as exposure to ionomycin for a longer time produces inferior proliferation of NK cells.

H. JAM test[5]

Materials and reagents

- RPMI 1640 medium with 5% FCS
- 96-well, flat- or round-bottom tissue culture plates (Costar)
- 24-well tissue culture plates (Costar)
- Scintillation vials
- Glass fiber filters
- 96-well harvester
- [^{3}H-methyl] thymidine (Amersham)
- Liquid scintillation counter
- Humidified 37°C, 5% CO_2 incubator

Protocol

1. Label target cells with [^{3}H-methyl] thymidine as follows: Add [^{3}H-methyl] thymidine to a final concentration of 2.5 to 5 μCi/ml (9.25 to 18.5×10^4 Bq/ml) to growing target cells (concentration 2.5 to 5×10^5 cells/ml) in 24-well tissue culture plates and incubate for 4 to 6 hr. Wash the cells once in RPMI 1640 medium with 5% FCS and resuspend to 1×10^5 cells/ml.
2. Dilute effector cells to an appropriate concentration depending on the experimental design. It is recommended to use three different effector:target ratios. The actual ratio used is dependent on factors such as target sensitivity and the effector cell potency.
3. Add 100 μl of effector cells into wells of the 96-well plates in triplicate. Leave row A empty.
4. Add 100 μl medium into the first three wells of row A for spontaneous death control.
5. Add 100 μl of [^{3}H-methyl] thymidine-labeled target cells to each well containing effector cells and to the second three wells of row A (maximum lysis control).
6. Incubate the plate for 2 hr in a humidified 37°C, 5% CO_2 incubator.
7. Add 100 μl of 2% SDS into those wells for maximum lysis control (second three wells, row A).

8. Aspirate the cells and their medium onto glass fiber filters using a cell harvester (normally used for harvesting cells for proliferation assay; see Chapter 3), wash the filters dry, add liquid scintillation fluid, and count in a liquid scintillation counter.
9. Calculation:

$$\% \text{ Specific DNA loss} = \frac{(T-E)-(T-S)}{T-(T-S)} \times 100$$

where E = experimentally retained DNA in the presence of NK cells; S = retained DNA in the absence of NK cells (spontaneous), and T = total incorporated label (maximum).

References

1. Sanderson, A.R., Cytotoxic reaction of mouse isoantisera: preliminary consideration, *Br. J. Exp. Pathol.*, 45, 398, 1964.
2. Brunner, K.T., Mauel, J., Cerottini, J.C., and Chapuis, B., Quantitative assay of the lytic action of immune lymphoid cells on ^{51}Cr-labelled allogeneic target cells *in vitro*; inhibition by isoantibody and by drugs, *Immunology*, 14, 181, 1968.
3. Gorer, P.A. and O'Gorman, P., The cytotoxic activity of isoantibodies in mice, *Transpl. Bull.*, 3, 142, 1956.
4. Duke, R.C., Chervenak, R., and Cohen, J.J., Endogenous endonuclease-induced DNA fragmentation: an early event in cell-mediated cytolysis, *Proc. Natl. Acad. Sci. U.S.A.*, 80, 6361, 1983.
5. Matzinger, P., The JAM test. A simple assay for DNA fragmentation and cell death, *J. Immunol. Methods*, 145, 185, 1991.
6. Nelson, D.L., Kurman, C.C., and Serbousek, D.E., ^{51}Cr release assay of antibody-dependent cell-mediated cytotoxicity (ADCC), in, *Current Protocols in Immunology*, Colignan, J.E., Kruisbeek, A.M., Margulies, D.H., Shevach, E.M., and Strober, W., Eds., Greene Publishing and Wiley InterScience, New York, 1991, 7.27.1.
7. Korzeniewski, C. and Callewaert, D.M., An enzyme-release assay for natural cytotoxicity, *J. Immunol. Methods*, 64, 313, 1983.
8. Decker, T. and Lohmann-Matthes, M.L., A quick and simple method for the quantitation of lactate dehydrogenase release in measurements of cellular cytotoxicity and tumor necrosis factor (TNF) activity, *J. Immunol. Methods*, 115, 61, 1988.
9. Timonen, T., Reynolds, C.W., Ortaldo, J.R., and Herberman, R.B., Isolation of human and rat natural killer cells, *J. Immunol. Methods*, 51, 269, 1982
10. Robertson, M.J., Manley, T.J., Donahue, C., Levine, H., and Ritz, J., Costimulatory signals are required for ptimal proliferation of human natural killer cells, *J. Immunol.*, 150, 1705, 1993.

chapter six

Assays of cytokines

Contents

I. Introduction

Cytokines are a group of small glycoproteins (~15 to 45 kDa) whose main function is to act as intercellular signals. Cytokines are secreted by and act on lymphocytes, monocyte/macrophages, and a variety of other cells, including cells of nonhemopoietic origin. Although many physiologic processes are regulated by cytokines, the regulation of inflammatory and immunologic responses are two of their main functions.[1] More than 100 different cytokines have been identified and their genes cloned.[2]

In most cases, the synthesis of cytokines is not constitutive but inducible by a variety of stimuli, depending on the nature of the secreting cell. In the case of lymphocytes, immunological stimulation by antigens or mitogens is the main trigger of cytokine secretion, whereas endotoxin and other microbial components are the main substances that induce cytokine synthesis and release from monocytes and other inflammatory cells.[3] Thus, because cytokine synthesis is a consequence of cellular activation, the *in vitro* or *in vivo* assessment of cytokine synthesis has been commonly used as a parameter of cellular activation. In addition, because different cell types and even different cell subsets secrete different sets of cytokines (i.e., Th1 and Th2 subsets of $CD4^+$ T cells),[4,5] the identification and quantification of cytokines allow the study of particular cell types or subsets activated by a particular signal or during a particular pathologic process.

Although the measurement of cytokines is well-established at the levels of basic and experimental immunology, evidence has indicated that cytokine assays may also have significant clinical value, particularly for prognostic or monitoring purposes.[6] Whether for research or clinical purposes, cytokine expression, synthesis, and secretion can be investigated by a variety of different techniques, including:

1. Assay of secreted cytokines in supernatants or biological fluids
2. Analysis of expression of cytokine-specific mRNA by Northern blotting, ribonuclease protection assays (RPA), or reverse-transcriptase polymerase chain reaction (RT-PCR)
3. Detection of cytokines in tissue samples by immunohistochemistry or *in situ* hybridization
4. Intracellular cytokine staining and flow cytometry
5. Detection of cytokine-secreting cells by ELISPOT assays

The subject of this chapter is the assay of secreted cytokines. Assays for cytokine RNA expression and intracellular cytokine staining are described elsewhere.[7]

A. *Assay of secreted cytokines*

The concentration of different cytokines present in biological fluids (e.g., serum, plasma, urine, saliva) or in tissue culture supernatants can be determined based on their biological activity (Section II) or on their immunogenicity or receptor-binding properties (Section III). These two different techniques have inherent advantages and disadvantages that need to be taken into consideration depending on the purpose of the cytokine measurement. Both types of assays are discussed in this chapter.

B. Standardization of cytokine measurements

All cytokine assays — whether bioassays or immunoassays — require the use of standard preparations of recombinant cytokines of known activity and concentration. Although many human and murine cytokines are available from commercial sources and these preparations can be routinely used as standards, cytokine assays should be calibrated against reference cytokine preparations. Reference standards are available from the Biological Response Modifiers Program (BRMP), National Cancer Institute (Frederick, MD), and the Division of Microbiology and Infectious Diseases, National Institute for Allergy and Infectious Diseases (NIAID, Bethesda, MD) in the U.S.; and from the National Institute for Biological Standards and Control (NIBSC) in London, U.K. These reagents are provided in small amounts for calibration or standard purposes only and are defined in terms of units of biological activity (U/ml). Although many commercially available cytokine preparations and ELISA kits are based on cytokine concentration expressed in terms of weight units per milliliter (e.g., ng/ml), reference standards can be used to calibrate the specific activity (e.g., Units/ng) of such preparations.

II. Bioassays

Before the availability of large amounts of recombinant cytokines and monoclonal anti-cytokine antibodies, cytokines were identified and assayed based on their biological activity, normally using *indicator cells*, which could be either freshly isolated cells or established cell lines. Although bioassays are still a convenient way to identify and/or quantify cytokines, it has become evident that most indicator cells are seldom cytokine-specific and can usually respond to several other cytokines in addition to the one they are intended to measure.[6] Hence, specificity may be a problem. For example, HT-2 or CTLL cell lines, which had been extensively used for the measurement of IL-2,[8,9] were later found to respond also to IL-4[10] and more recently to IL-15.[11] Nevertheless, when used in conjunction with appropriate neutralizing anti-cytokine monoclonal antibodies to either confirm the identity of the cytokine being measured or to neutralize potentially interfering cytokines, bioassays still offer relatively simple and sensitive means for cytokine assay. The main advantages and disadvantages of bioassays are listed below.

Advantages

1. Measure only "functional" cytokines (true reflection of biological activity)
2. Very sensitive (~10 pg/ml)
3. Relatively inexpensive

Disadvantages

1. Indicator cells are usually not cytokine-specific (may respond to more than one cytokine and may be susceptible to synergistic or inhibitory effects of other cytokines)
2. Susceptible to inhibitors (e.g., cytokine antagonists, soluble cytokine receptors) present in biological fluids
3. Do not differentiate between subtypes of cytokines (e.g., IL-1α and IL-1β, TNFα and TNFβ, etc.)
4. Reproducibility may be compromised due to variability in indicator cells
5. Lengthy (results may take from one to several days)

Although there could be as many different bioassays as different cytokines, most are based on:

1. *Proliferation*: measurement of proliferative response of indicator cell lines in response to the appropriate cytokine. Usually performed by assessing tritiated thymidine uptake or MTT-reduction (see Chapter 3).
2. *Cytotoxicity*: based on the cytotoxicity of certain cytokines for appropriate indicator cell lines or on protection from viral infection and lysis. Usually performed by assessing inhibition of cellular proliferation, ^{51}Cr release, or decreased cell viability.
3. *Differentiation*: based on the induction of a differentiation function on a target cell. These could include expression of surface molecules, including MHC class I and II molecules; secretion of immunoglobulins, including different isotypes; formation of colonies on soft agar, etc.

In conclusion, cytokine bioassays can provide a very useful way of measuring cytokines as long as adequate precautions are taken to ensure their specificity (i.e., through neutralizing anti-cytokine monoclonal antibodies). Bioassays for the most commonly assayed cytokines are described below. Note that although most of the protocols for bioassays based on proliferation assays are performed by tritiated thymidine uptake, these can also be adapted to an MTT-reduction assay (see Chapter 3). Immunoassays are described later in this chapter.

A. *Interleukin-1*

Interleukin-1 (IL-1) is an extremely pleiotropic cytokine secreted by cells of the monocyte/macrophage lineage and many other types of cells of lymphocytic, myeloid, and nonhemopoietic origin.[12] IL-1 plays a key role as a mediator of inflammation and has important activities promoting activation and differentiation of T and B lymphocytes.[2,12] In humans and mice, IL-1 exists in two different forms, IL-1α and IL-1β, encoded by different genes sharing only moderate sequence homology.[2,12] Both IL-1α and IL-1β are synthesized as large cytoplasmic precursors that are proteolytically processed and released as the mature forms.[2,12] In addition to secreted IL-1, membrane-bound IL-1 activity has been reported in fixed cells.[13] Two different receptors for IL-1 (type I and type II IL-1R) have been identified.[14,15] Moreover, the activity of IL-1 *in vivo* appears to be regulated by an endogenous IL-1 receptor antagonist (IL-1Ra), a molecule that exhibits approximately 26% sequence homology with IL-1β and is able to bind to IL-1Rs without triggering any biologic activity.[16]

Many different bioassays for IL-1 have been described, including the co-stimulatory activity on thymocytes[17] and the D10.G4.1 T cell line,[18] induction of IL-2 secretion from the lymphoma cell lines LRBM.33.1A5[19] or EL-4,[20] proliferation of fibroblasts,[21] and inhibition of the proliferation of the A375 human malignant melanoma cell line.[22] The first two assays are described in this chapter. Because human IL-1 is active on murine systems, both human and murine IL-1 can be assayed using either protocol.

1. Thymocyte co-stimulation assay

This assay is based on the ability of IL-1 to potentiate the proliferation of murine thymocytes in response to phytohemagglutinin (PHA). This assay does not differentiate between IL-1α and IL-1β activities.

Materials and reagents

- Mouse (C3H/HeJ) thymocyte suspension
- Culture medium: RPMI-1640 containing 10% heat-inactivated FCS and supplemented with 2 m*M* L-glutamine, 10 m*M* HEPES, 100 U/ml penicillin, 100 μg/ml streptomycin, 50 μ*M* 2-mercaptoethanol, and 1 m*M* sodium pyruvate
- Washing buffer: PBS containing 1% FCS (filter-sterilized)
- Phytohemagglutinin-P (PHA, Sigma Cat. No. L-9132)
- Recombinant human or mouse IL-1 standard (e.g., BD Pharmingen, Biosource International, Endogen)
- [^{3}H-methyl] thymidine
- 96-well tissue culture plates (flat bottom), sterile
- 15- and 50-ml centrifuge tubes
- 60 × 15-mm Petri dishes
- Pasteur pipettes
- Refrigerated centrifuge (set at 4°C)
- CO_2 incubator (humidified, set at 37°C and 5% CO_2)
- Cell harvester (e.g., Skatron)
- Glass fiber filter mats (Skatron)
- Scintillation vials
- Scintillation cocktail (e.g., Econo-Safe™, Research Products International)
- Scintillation counter

Protocol

(*Note*: All materials and reagents must be sterile and proper aseptic techniques must be used when handling the cells.)

1. Sacrifice the animal and prepare a thymocyte suspension (Chapter 1) by removing the thymus, rinsing it in a 60 × 15-mm Petri dish with 10 ml washing buffer, and then grinding it with the aid of two sterile, frosted glass slides in another sterile Petri dish containing 10 ml ice-cold washing buffer.
2. Collect the cell suspension and transfer it to a 50-ml centrifuge tube with a sterile Pasteur pipette. Wash the cells once by resuspending them in 50 ml washing buffer and centrifuge for 10 min at 200*g* in a refrigerated (4°C) centrifuge.
3. Aspirate the supernatant and resuspend the cells in culture medium. Count. Adjust cell density with culture medium to a cell density of 10^7 cells/ml.
4. Determine the number of wells required. Each sample and standard dilution should be assayed in triplicate. In addition, include a negative control in which the thymocytes are cultured with no added source of IL-1. (A minimum of six or seven different dilutions of the IL-1 standard should be tested.)
5. Add 100 μl thymocyte suspension per well. Add 50 μl of a (4X) PHA solution made in culture medium. (The final concentration of PHA in the cultures should be determined beforehand. For this, first test several concentrations of PHA [0.1 to 5 μg/ml] and choose a concentration giving suboptimal proliferation and maximal enhancement by an rIL-1 standard.)
6. Add samples and rIL-1 standards (1 to 1000 pg/ml) diluted in culture medium. Each dilution should be assayed in triplicate. Incubate for 48 hr at 37°C and 5% CO_2.
7. Add 20 μl/well of a 50-μCi/ml solution of [^{3}H-methyl] thymidine in culture medium (final concentration is 1 μCi/well) for the last 6 hr of incubation.
8. Harvest the cells onto glass fiber mats with the aid of a cell harvester. Determine [^{3}H-methyl] thymidine uptake by liquid scintillation counting (see Chapter 3).
9. Calculate the IL-1 concentration. Using semilog or probit paper, plot standard IL-1 concentration on the x-axis vs. proliferation (in cpm) on the y-axis. Calculate sample concentration by comparison to a standard curve and multiplication by dilution factor.

Comments

1. Although thymocytes from other strains are also responsive to IL-1, thymocytes from C3H/HeJ mice are generally used in this assay due

to their high responsiveness. The use of animals 6 to 12 weeks old is recommended.

2. When assaying unknown samples, test several dilutions so that a curve for those samples can be generated. Concentrations can then be calculated by comparison of sample dilution giving 50% maximal response with the standard concentration giving 50% maximal proliferation. For example:

$$\text{Sample concentration} = \text{Standard concentration (50\% max)} \times \text{Sample dilution (50\% max)}$$

3. Several other cytokines, including IL-2, IL-6, and TNFα, may also induce proliferation of thymocytes in the presence of mitogen.

2. Co-stimulation assay using the D10.G4.1 cell line

This assay is based on the ability of IL-1 to stimulate the proliferation of the T helper cell line D10.G4.1 in the presence of a suboptimal concentration of Concanavalin A. D10.G4.1 is a murine $CD4^+$ T cell clone with specificity for conalbumin presented by accessory cells expressing the $I\text{-}A^k$ MHC class II molecule.[23] This assay does not differentiate between IL-1α and IL-1β activities.

Materials and reagents

- D10.G4.1 cells (ATCC Cat. No. TIB 224)
- Concanavalin A (ConA; Sigma Cat. No. C-5275)
- Culture medium: RPMI-1640 containing 10% heat-inactivated FCS and supplemented with 2 m*M* L-glutamine, 10 m*M* HEPES, 100 U/ml penicillin, 100 μg/ml streptomycin, 50 μ*M* 2-mercaptoethanol, and 1 m*M* sodium pyruvate
- Washing buffer: PBS containing 1% FCS (filter-sterilized)
- Recombinant human or mouse IL-1 standard (e.g., BD Pharmingen, Biosource International, Endogen)
- [^{3}H-methyl] thymidine
- 96-well tissue culture plates (flat bottom), sterile
- 15- and 50-ml centrifuge tubes
- Pasteur pipettes
- Refrigerated centrifuge (set at 4°C)
- CO_2 incubator (humidified, set at 37°C and 5% CO_2)
- Cell harvester (e.g., Skatron)
- Glass fiber filter mats (Skatron)
- Scintillation vials

- Scintillation cocktail (e.g., Econo-Safe™, Research Products International)
- Scintillation counter

Protocol

(*Note*: All materials and reagents must be sterile and proper aseptic techniques must be used when handling the cells.)

1. Harvest the D10.G4.1 cells approximately 7 days after the last stimulation (see maintenance of D10.G4.1 cells). Wash the cells 2× in 20 ml ice-cold washing buffer, centrifuging at 200*g* at a temperature of 4°C. Resuspend cells in culture medium containing 2.5 μg/ml ConA to a cell density of 10^5 cells/ml.
2. Determine the number of wells required. Each sample and standard dilution should be assayed in triplicate. In addition, include a negative control, in which the D10.G4.1 cells are cultured with no added source of IL-1. (A minimum of six or seven different dilutions of the IL-1 standard [1 to 1000 pg/ml] should be tested.)
3. Add 100 μl of the cell suspension per well.
4. Add test samples and standards diluted in culture medium (100 μl/well). Assay each dilution in triplicate.
5. Incubate for 72 hr at 37°C and 5% CO_2. Add 20 μl/well of a 50-μCi/ml solution of [^{3}H-methyl] thymidine in culture medium (final concentration is 1 μCi/well) for the last 6 hr of incubation.
6. Harvest the cells onto glass fiber filters with the aid of a cell harvester. Determine [^{3}H-methyl] thymidine uptake by liquid scintillation counting (see Chapter 3).
7. Calculate the IL-1 concentration. Using semilog or probit paper, plot standard IL-1 concentration on the *x*-axis vs. proliferation (in cpm) on the *y*-axis. Calculate the sample concentration by comparison to standard curve and multiplication by dilution factor.

3. Maintenance of D10.G4.1 cells

Materials and reagents

- Spleen cells from mice expressing I-A^k MHC class II (e.g., AKR, CBA/J, C3H/HeJ)
- Mitomycin C (Sigma Cat. No. M-0503)
- Conalbumin (Sigma Cat. No. C-0755)
- Recombinant human or murine IL-2 (rIL-2) (e.g., Genzyme)
- Culture medium: RPMI-1640 containing 10% heat-inactivated FCS and supplemented with 2 m*M* L-glutamine, 10 m*M* HEPES, 100

U/ml penicillin, 100 μg/ml streptomycin, 50 μ*M* 2-mercaptoethanol, and 1 m*M* sodium pyruvate
- Washing buffer: PBS containing 1% FCS (filter-sterilized)
- 24-well tissue culture plates or 100 × 15-mm Petri dishes
- 60 × 15-mm Petri dishes
- 15- and 50-ml centrifuge tubes
- Pasteur pipettes
- Refrigerated centrifuge (set at 4°C)
- CO_2 incubator (humidified, set at 37°C and 5% CO_2)
- Sterile forceps

Protocol

(*Note*: All materials and reagents must be sterile and proper aseptic techniques must be used when handling the cells.)

1. Sacrifice mice and aseptically remove the spleens. Wash the spleens in a 60 × 15-mm Petri dish with 10 ml ice-cold washing buffer and prepare a splenic cell suspension by gently teasing the spleens with a pair of sterile forceps. Wash the cells 2× with 40 ml cold washing buffer.
2. Resuspend the cells in culture medium to a cell density of 2×10^7 cells/ml. Add mitomycin C to a final concentration of 50 μg/ml and incubate in a 37°C water bath for 30 to 60 min with occasional agitation. Wash the cells 4× with washing buffer. Count and resuspend in culture medium to a density of 1×10^7 cells/ml.
3. Using 24-well tissue culture plates, 100 × 15-mm Petri dishes, or tissue culture flasks (depending on the number of cells and volume of medium), culture the D10.G4.1 cells at 37°C, 5% CO_2 and a final density of 1 to 2×10^5/ml in the presence of mitomycin C-treated splenic cells (final density of 5×10^6/ml), conalbumin (100 μg/ml), and rIL-2 (100 U/ml). Repeat this stimulation every 2 weeks. Passage the cells at a 1:5 dilution in IL-2-containing medium (100 U/ml) if the culture medium becomes yellow.

Comments

1. IL-2 may mimic IL-1 in this assay.
2. Conditioned medium from ConA-activated splenocytes can be used as a source of IL-2 (instead of the rIL-2) for the maintenance of the D10.G4.1 cells. To prepare the conditioned medium, prepare a splenic cell suspension from BALB/c mice and culture at 10^7 cells/ml in the presence of ConA (5 μg/ml) for 24 hr at 37°C and 5% CO_2. Collect the supernatant by centrifugation, filter, and store at –20°C until use. Use at 5 to 10% final concentration.

B. Interleukin-2

Interleukin-2 (IL-2) is a cytokine produced by activated $CD4^+$ and some $CD8^+$ T lymphocytes.[4,24] In addition to being the major T cell growth factor for both human and murine T cells, IL-2 also stimulates growth and differentiation of cytotoxic T cell precursors (CTLs), growth and cytotoxic activity of NK cells, proliferation and differentiation of activated human B cells, and activation of monocytes.[2,24] The biological effects of IL-2 are mediated by binding to high-affinity IL-2 receptors (IL-2Rs), which are composed of at least three different subunits: IL-2Rα (CD25, p55, Tac antigen), IL-2Rβ (CD122, p75), and IL-2Rγ (CD132, γ_c).[25] Signaling through the IL-2R requires the γ_c chain, which is also shared with other cytokine receptors, including IL-4R, IL-7R, and IL-15R.[26-29] Upon activation, T cells also release truncated forms of the α-subunit, which appear as soluble IL-2Rs in supernatants or biological fluids.[30]

The bioassays for IL-2 are all based on its ability to stimulate the proliferation of murine T cell lines, such as HT-2 and CTLL-2.[7,8] These cell lines respond to and can be used to assay both human and murine IL-2. However, because murine IL-4 also stimulates the proliferation of both HT-2 and CTLL-2 cells,[10] assays involving mouse-derived samples need to be performed in the presence of neutralizing anti-mouse IL-4 antibodies to make the assay monospecific for IL-2. Conversely, performing the proliferation assay in the presence of neutralizing anti-mouse IL-2 antibodies makes the assay specific for IL-4. Human IL-4 is not active in murine systems, and thus no blocking anti-human IL-4 antibodies are required for the human IL-2 assay.

1. HT-2 or CTLL-2 proliferation assay for IL-2/IL-4

This assay, which is routinely used to measure IL-2 and/or IL-4, is based on the proliferation of the IL-2/IL-4-responsive T cell lines, HT-2[8] or CTLL-2.[9]

Materials and reagents

- Indicator cells: HT-2 (ATCC Cat. No. CRL 1841) or CTLL-2 cells (ATCC Cat. No. TIB 214)
- Recombinant human or mouse IL-2 standard
- Recombinant mouse IL-4 standard
- Rat monoclonal anti-mouse IL-4 (11B11) (ATCC Cat. No. HB 188)
- Rat monoclonal anti-mouse IL-2 (S4B6) (ATCC Cat. No. HB 8794)
- Recombinant human or murine IL-2 (rIL-2) (e.g., BD Pharmingen, Biosource International, Endogen)
- Culture medium: RPMI-1640 containing 10% heat-inactivated FCS and supplemented with 2 m*M* L-glutamine, 10 m*M* HEPES, 100 U/ml penicillin, 100 μg/ml streptomycin, 50 μ*M* 2-mercaptoethanol, and 1 m*M* sodium pyruvate

- Washing buffer: PBS containing 1% FCS (filter-sterilized)
- [^{3}H-methyl] thymidine
- 96-well tissue culture plates (flat bottom)
- 15- and 50-ml centrifuge tubes
- Pasteur pipettes
- Refrigerated centrifuge (set at 4°C)
- CO_2 incubator (humidified, set at 37°C and 5% CO_2)
- Cell harvester (e.g., Skatron)
- Glass fiber filter mats (Skatron)
- Scintillation vials
- Scintillation cocktail (e.g., Econo-Safe™, Research Products International)
- Scintillation counter

Protocol

(*Note*: All materials and reagents must be sterile and proper aseptic techniques must be used when handling the cells.)

1. Harvest the indicator cells, usually at the end of the second or third day of culture (see maintenance of HT-2 and CTLL-2 cells below), and wash twice with 20 ml cold washing buffer and once with complete medium to remove any IL-2. Determine viability by Trypan blue exclusion and count. Resuspend the cells in culture medium to a cell density of 2.5×10^5 cells/ml. Maintain the cells in an ice bath until use.
2. Dilute samples and standards (10 to 10,000 pg/ml) in culture medium. Assay each dilution in triplicate. Include a background proliferation control in which the indicator cells are cultured in the presence of medium alone. Normally, six to seven different dilutions of the standard are required for the standard curve.
3. Add 20 to 50 µl of sample or recombinant IL-2/IL-4 standard per well.
4. If it is unknown whether samples contain IL-2, IL-4, or both, neutralizing anti-IL-2 or anti-IL-4 antibodies need to be included. Prepare one set of samples without antibodies, another with anti-IL-2 monoclonal antibody (S4B6, usually at a final concentration of 10 µg/ml), and another with anti-IL-4 monoclonal antibody (11B11, again at 10 µg/ml). Pre-incubate samples and antibodies for 30 min at room temperature.
5. Add enough culture medium to bring the volume of each well to 80 µl.
6. Add 20 µl indicator cell suspension to each well (5000 cells/well). The final volume is 100 µl. Incubate for 24 hr at 37°C in a 5% CO_2 atmosphere.
7. Add 20 µl/well of a 50 µCi/ml solution of [^{3}H-methyl] thymidine in culture medium (final concentration is 1 µCi/well). Incubate overnight at 37°C and 5% CO_2.

8. Harvest the cells onto glass fiber mats with the aid of a cell harvester. Determine [^{3}H-methyl] thymidine uptake by liquid scintillation counting (see Chapter 3).
9. Calculate IL-2 (wells containing anti-IL-4 antibodies) and/or IL-4 concentrations (wells containing anti-IL-2 antibodies) by reference to recombinant IL-2 and IL-4 standards, respectively. Using semilog or probit paper, plot standard IL-2/4 concentration on the *x*-axis vs. proliferation (in cpm) on the *y*-axis. Calculate the sample concentration by comparison to standard curve and multiplication by dilution factor.

2. Maintenance of HT-2 or CTLL-2 cells

Materials and reagents

- HT-2 (ATCC Cat. CRL 1841) or CTLL-2 cells (ATCC Cat. No. TIB 214)
- Culture medium: RPMI-1640 containing 10% heat-inactivated FCS and supplemented with 2 m*M* L-glutamine, 10 m*M* HEPES, 100 U/ml penicillin, 100 μg/ml streptomycin, 50 μ*M* 2-mercaptoethanol, and 1 m*M* sodium pyruvate
- Recombinant IL-2 (human or mouse)
- 25-cm^2 culture flasks
- 15- and 50-ml centrifuge tubes
- Pasteur pipettes
- Refrigerated centrifuge (set at 4°C)
- CO_2 incubator (humidified, set at 37°C and 5% CO_2)

Protocol

(*Note*: All materials and reagents must be sterile and proper aseptic techniques must be used when handling the cells.)

1. Seed HT-2 or CTLL-2 cells at an initial density of 1×10^5 cells/ml in culture medium containing rIL-2 (10 to 20 U/ml).
2. Culture at 37°C and 5% CO_2 for 3 days. At this point, the cells can be harvested and used in the IL-2/IL-4 assay.
3. Subculture every third day.

Comments

1. It is recommended to use only indicator cells with >90% viability after harvesting.
2. Although these cell lines proliferate in response to murine IL-4, they cannot be maintained for long periods of time exclusively in IL-4.
3. CTLL-2 cells also proliferate in response to IL-15.[11]
4. Conditioned medium from ConA-activated splenocytes can also be used as a source of IL-2 for maintenance of HT-2 or CTLL-2 cell lines (refer to Section A.3 in this chapter for preparation).

C. Interleukin-3

Interleukin-3 (IL-3), also known as multi-colony stimulating factor (Multi-CSF) or mast cell growth factor, is a cytokine produced primarily by activated T lymphocytes, myelomonocytic cell lines (WEHI-3), and activated mast cells and NK cells.[4,31,32] IL-3 is a member of a group of cytokines whose main function is to promote the growth and differentiation of hemopoietic precursor cells. In particular, IL-3 acts on pluripotent bone marrow stem cells to induce the generation of all types of hemopoietic colonies (granulocytes, monocytes, megakaryocytes, mast cells, eosinophils) in soft agar.[33] In addition, IL-3 stimulates the growth of mast cell lines and potentiates the activities of eosinophils, basophils, and mast cells.[34] The effects of IL-3 are mediated through binding to high-affinity IL-3 receptors (IL-3Rs), which are heterodimers formed by an α-chain (CD123, 70 kDa) that binds IL-3, and by a signal-transducing β-subunit (CD131, 130 kDa, β_c) that is shared among IL-3, GM-CSF, and IL-5 receptors.[35,36]

Although IL-3 and other colony-stimulating factors, such as GM-CSF, G-CSF, and M-CSF, can be assayed based on their activity inducing the formation of hemopoietic colonies in soft agar,[33] the availability of IL-3-dependent mast cell and myeloid cell lines, including FDCP-2,[37] FD.C/1,[38] 32D,[39] and MC/9,[40] has made it possible to assay IL-3 based on simple proliferation assays such as those already described for IL-2 and IL-4. Because human and murine IL-3 are species specific in their actions, the indicator cell lines mentioned above (all of murine origin) are suitable only for the assay of mouse IL-3. However, human IL-3 can be assayed using the IL-3-responsive erythroleukemia cell line, TF-1.[41]

1. IL-3-dependent cell line proliferation assay

Materials and reagents

- IL-3-dependent cell line: MC/9 (mouse, ATCC Cat. No. CRL-8306); TF-1 (human, ATCC Cat. No. CRL-2003)
- Recombinant IL-3 standard (mouse or human)
- Culture medium: RPMI-1640 containing 10% heat-inactivated FCS and supplemented with 2 m*M* L-glutamine, 10 m*M* HEPES, 100 U/ml penicillin, 100 μg/ml streptomycin, 50 μ*M* 2-mercaptoethanol, and 1 m*M* sodium pyruvate
- Washing buffer: PBS containing 1% FCS (filter-sterilized)
- [^{3}H-methyl] thymidine
- 96-well tissue culture plates (flat bottom)
- 15- and 50-ml centrifuge tubes
- Pasteur pipettes
- Refrigerated centrifuge (set at 4°C)
- CO_2 incubator (humidified, set at 37°C and 5% CO_2)
- Cell harvester (e.g., Skatron)

- Glass fiber filter mats (Skatron)
- Scintillation vials
- Scintillation cocktail (e.g., Econo-Safe™, Research Products International)
- Scintillation counter

Protocol

(*Note*: All materials and reagents must be sterile and proper aseptic techniques must be used when handling the cells.)

1. Harvest indicator cells and wash twice with cold washing buffer and once with culture medium to remove any IL-3. Count and resuspend the cells to a density of 5×10^4 cells/ml in culture medium.
2. Dilute test samples and standards (0.1 to 100 U/ml) in culture medium. Include a negative control (background proliferation) containing medium only. Plate at 100 μl per well (in triplicate).
3. Add 100 μl of the indicator cell suspension to each well (final: 5000 cells/well).
4. Incubate the plate for 24 hr at 37°C and 5% CO_2.
5. Add 20 μl/well of a 50-μCi/ml solution of [^{3}H-methyl] thymidine in culture medium (final concentration is 1 μCi/well). Incubate overnight at 37°C and 5% CO_2.
6. Harvest the cells onto glass fiber filters with the aid of a cell harvester. Determine [^{3}H-methyl] thymidine uptake by liquid scintillation counting.
7. Calculate the IL-3 concentration by reference to recombinant IL-3. Using semilog or probit paper, plot standard IL-3 concentration on the *x*-axis vs. proliferation (in cpm) on the *y*-axis. Calculate the sample concentration by comparison to standard curve and multiplication by dilution factor.

2. Maintenance of IL-3-dependent cell lines

Materials and reagents

- IL-3-dependent cell line: MC/9 (mouse, ATCC Cat. No. CRL-8306); TF-1 (human, ATCC Cat. No. CRL-2003)
- Recombinant IL-3 (mouse or human, depending on origin of indicator cell line) or recombinant GM-CSF (human)
- Culture medium: RPMI-1640 containing 10% heat-inactivated FCS and supplemented with 2 m*M* L-glutamine, 10 m*M* HEPES, 100 U/ml penicillin, 100 μg/ml streptomycin, 50 μM 2-mercaptoethanol, and 1 m*M* sodium pyruvate
- Washing buffer: PBS containing 1% FCS (filter-sterilized)
- 25-cm^2 culture flasks
- 15- and 50-ml centrifuge tubes

- Pasteur pipettes
- Refrigerated centrifuge (set at 4°C)
- CO_2 incubator (humidified, set at 37°C and 5% CO_2)

Protocol

(*Note*: All materials and reagents must be sterile and proper aseptic techniques must be used when handling the cells.)

1. Seed cells at an initial density of 1×10^5 cells/ml in culture medium containing rIL-3 (50 to 100 U/ml). TF-1 cells have been maintained in culture medium containing 1 ng/ml recombinant human GM-CSF.[28]
2. Culture at 37°C and 5% CO_2 for 3 days. At this point, the cells can be harvested and used in the IL-3 assay.
3. Subculture every third day.

Comments

1. Immune complexes and aggregated immunoglobulins stimulate mast cell lines by binding to their Fc receptors, inducing the production of cytokines (including IL-3) and proliferation[41]
2. Conditioned medium from the myelomonocytic cell line WEHI-3 (ATCC Cat. No. TIB 68) can be used as a source of murine IL-3. To prepare, culture WEHI-3 cells at 10^6 cells/ml in culture medium for 48 hr at 37°C and 5% CO_2. Collect supernatant by centrifugation and filter. Aliquot and store at –20°C. Use at a final concentration of 5 to 10%.
3. The human erythroleukemia cell line (TF-1),[41] is responsive to and has been used to assay for IL-5 and GM-CSF. The use of appropriate neutralizing antibodies is required to confirm specificity.

D. *Interleukin-4*

Interleukin-4 (IL-4) is a highly pleiotropic cytokine secreted by a subset of $CD4^+$ T cells (Th2) and mast cells.[43,44] IL-4 has many important activities, including MHC class II molecule and CD23 expression on B cells, the induction of isotype class switch (IgG_1, IgE) in B lymphocytes,[45,46] the proliferation and maturation of activated $CD4^+$ T lymphocytes into the IL-4/IL-5/IL-10-secreting (Th2) subset,[47-49] growth of mast cell lines, activation of some monocytic cell functions, and inhibition of expression of inflammatory cytokines by monocytes.[43,50] IL-4 exerts its effects by interacting with high-affinity IL-4 receptors, which are present on a wide variety of hemopoietic and nonhemopoietic cell types.[51-53] The functional IL-4R has been shown to be composed of a 140-kDa IL-4-binding subunit[54-56] (CD124) in noncovalent association with the cytokine receptor common γ_c chain (IL-2Rγ, CD132),[26,27] which is shared with other cytokine receptors, including IL-2R,[26,27] IL-7R,[28] IL-13R,[29] and IL-15R.[11] In addition to the membrane-bound form, soluble IL-4R forms are also synthesized and released into biological fluids.[54,57]

A wide variety of bioassays have been established for the measurement of IL-4, based on its many activities. Some of these assays include the increased expression of MHC class II molecules on B cells,[58] proliferation of B cells stimulated with anti-immunoglobulin antibodies,[59] secretion of IgG_1 or IgE by lipopolysaccharide (LPS)-stimulated B lymphocytes,[60,61] and proliferation of IL-4-responsive T cell and mast cell lines.[10,40] Human and murine IL-4 are species specific in their action. The most commonly used and simple bioassays for murine IL-4 are proliferation assays using IL-4/IL-2-responsive T cell lines, such as HT-2[8] or CTLL-2[9] (described in Section B) or IL-4-responsive and relatively IL-2-unresponsive T cell lines such as CT.4S.[62] For the bioassay of human IL-4, murine T cell lines transfected with human IL-4Rs have been reported.[63]

1. CT.4S proliferation assay

The HT-2 or CTLL-2 proliferation assay for IL-2 and IL-4 was described in Section B of this chapter. This assay requires the inclusion of neutralizing monoclonal anti-IL-2 and anti-IL-4 to make the assay specific for IL-4 and IL-2, respectively. CT.4S cells, in contrast, exhibit high responsiveness to IL-4 while being unresponsive to IL-2, except at very high concentrations.[62] This assay is thus relatively specific for IL-4 (mouse) and does not require the use of neutralizing monoclonal anti-IL-4 antibodies. Nonetheless, as with all bioassays, it is always a good idea to confirm the specificity of the indicator cell line by inhibition with appropriate neutralizing antibodies.

Materials and reagents

- CT.4S cells
- Recombinant mouse IL-4 standard
- Culture medium: RPMI-1640 containing 10% heat-inactivated FCS and supplemented with 2 m*M* L-glutamine, 10 m*M* HEPES, 100 U/ml penicillin, 100 μg/ml streptomycin, 50 μ*M* 2-mercaptoethanol, and 1 m*M* sodium pyruvate
- Washing buffer: PBS containing 1% FCS (filter-sterilized)
- [^{3}H-methyl] thymidine
- 96-well tissue culture plates (flat bottom)
- 15- and 50-ml centrifuge tubes
- Pasteur pipettes
- Refrigerated centrifuge (set at 4°C)
- CO_2 incubator (humidified, set at 37°C and 5% CO_2)
- Cell harvester (e.g., Skatron)
- Glass fiber filter mats (Skatron)
- Scintillation vials

- Scintillation cocktail (e.g., Econo-Safe, Research Products International)
- Scintillation counter

Protocol

(*Note*: All materials and reagents must be sterile and proper aseptic techniques must be used when handling the cells.)

1. Dilute test samples and standards (10 to 10,000 pg/ml) in complete medium. Include a negative control containing medium only. Plate at 20 to 50 μl per well (in triplicate).
2. Add enough culture medium to bring the volume of each well to 80 μl.
3. Harvest the CT.4S cells, and wash twice with washing buffer and once with culture medium to remove any IL-4. Count and resuspend the cells to a density of 2.5×10^5 cells/ml in culture medium. It is advisable to harvest and prepare the indicator cell suspension just before its use.
4. Add 20 μl of the indicator cell suspension to each well (final: 5000 cells/well).
5. Incubate the plate for 24 hr at 37°C and 5% CO_2.
6. Add 20 μl/well of a 50 μCi/ml solution of [^{3}H-methyl] thymidine in culture medium (final concentration is 1 μCi/well). Incubate overnight at 37°C and 5% CO_2.
7. Harvest the cells onto glass fiber filters with the aid of a cell harvester. Determine [^{3}H-methyl] thymidine uptake by liquid scintillation counting.
8. Calculate IL-4 concentration by comparison to rIL-4 standard curve. Using semilog or probit paper, plot standard IL-4 concentration on the *x*-axis vs. proliferation (in cpm) on the *y*-axis. Calculate the sample concentration by comparison to standard curve and multiplication by dilution factor.

2. Maintenance of CT.4S cells

Materials and reagents

- CT.4S cells
- Recombinant IL-4 (mouse)
- Culture medium: RPMI-1640 containing 10% heat-inactivated FCS and supplemented with 2 m*M* L-glutamine, 10 m*M* HEPES, 100 U/ml penicillin, 100 μg/ml streptomycin, 50 μ*M* 2-mercaptoethanol, and 1 m*M* sodium pyruvate
- 25-cm^2 culture flasks
- 15- and 50-ml centrifuge tubes

- Pasteur pipettes
- Refrigerated centrifuge (set at 4°C)
- CO_2 incubator (humidified, set at 37°C and 5% CO_2)

Protocol

(*Note*: All materials and reagents must be sterile and proper aseptic techniques must be used when handling the cells.)

1. Seed cells at an initial density of 1×10^5 cells/ml in culture medium containing rIL-4 (5 to 10 ng/ml).
2. Culture at 37°C and 5% CO_2 for 3 days. At this point, the cells can be harvested by gently shaking the culture flask (cells are adherent) and used in the IL-4 assay.
3. Subculture every third day.

Comments

1. Murine T cell lines transfected with the human IL-4R (e.g., CTLL)[63] can be used for the bioassay of human IL-4 following a similar protocol, with the exception of human rIL-4 standards. Other bioassays for human IL-4 include the proliferation of human B cells stimulated with anti-IgM antibodies or *Staphylococcus aureus* Cowan strain I (SAC),[64] class II MHC molecule expression of the human Burkitt lymphoma cell line RAMOS (ATCC Cat. No. CRL 1596),[65] or proliferation of the erythroleukemia cell line TF-1.[41]

E. Interleukin-5

Interleukin-5 (IL-5) is a cytokine produced primarily by the Th2 subset of $CD4^+$ T cells.[4] Both in mice and humans, IL-5 appears to be the major cytokine responsible for eosinophilia, promoting the growth, differentiation, and activation of eosinophils.[66,67] In addition, murine IL-5 induces proliferation and differentiation of activated B lymphocytes, promotes immunoglobulin secretion, including IgA, and induces differentiation of thymocytes into CTLs.[68-70] Whether human IL-5 has similar effects on human B cells remains controversial. High-affinity receptors for IL-5 are heterodimers composed of an IL-5-binding subunit (CD125, IL-5Rα, 60 kDa) and a signal-transducing subunit (β_c, 130 kDa) shared with receptors for IL-3 and GM-CSF.[36]

A number of bioassays have been used for the measurement of IL-5, including co-stimulation with dextran sulfate on normal B lymphocytes,[68] proliferation of BCL_1 tumor cells,[71] and induction of IgM secretion by an *in vitro*-adapted clone of BCL_1 cells (BCL1 CW13.20-3B3).[69] Although BCL_1 cells are also reported to be sensitive to human IL-5, a much simpler proliferation assay using human erythroleukemia TF-1 cells (described in Section C)[41] can also be used for the measurement of human IL-5.

1. Dextran sulfate co-stimulation assay

Materials and reagents

- Splenic cell suspension from BALB/c mice
- Dextran sulfate (Sigma Cat. No. D-7037)
- Recombinant mouse IL-5 standard
- Culture medium: RPMI-1640 containing 10% heat-inactivated FCS and supplemented with 2 m*M* L-glutamine, 10 m*M* HEPES, 100 U/ml penicillin, 100 μg/ml streptomycin, 50 μ*M* 2-mercaptoethanol, and 1 m*M* sodium pyruvate
- Washing buffer: PBS containing 1% FCS (filter-sterilized)
- [^{3}H-methyl] thymidine
- 96-well tissue culture plates (flat bottom)
- 15- and 50-ml centrifuge tubes
- Pasteur pipettes
- Refrigerated centrifuge (set at 4°C)
- CO_2 incubator (humidified, set at 37°C and 5% CO_2)
- Cell harvester (e.g., Skatron)
- Glass fiber filter mats (Skatron)
- Scintillation vials
- Scintillation cocktail (e.g., Econo-Safe, Research Products International)
- Scintillation counter

Protocol

(*Note*: All materials and reagents must be sterile and proper aseptic techniques must be used when handling the cells.)

1. Sacrifice a BALB/c mouse by cervical dislocation and aseptically remove the spleen. Prepare a single cell suspension by gently teasing the spleen with a pair of sterile forceps or by forcing it through a wire-mesh screen. Collect the cell suspension (avoiding debris) and transfer it to a 50-ml centrifuge tube. Wash the cells 2× with 40 ml of cold washing buffer and centrifuge at 200*g* for 10 min. Count and resuspend in culture medium to a density of 1×10^6 cells/ml.
2. Dilute samples and standards (0.1 to 100 U/ml) in culture medium. Add 100 μl per well, including negative controls containing medium only. Set each dilution in triplicate.
3. Add 50 μl per well of an 80-μg/ml solution of dextran sulfate in culture medium.
4. Add 50 μl per well of the spleen cell suspension and incubate for 72 hr at 37°C and 5% CO_2.
5. Add 20 μl/well of a 50-μCi/ml solution of [^{3}H-methyl] thymidine in culture medium (final concentration is 1 μCi/well) during the last 18 hr of incubation.

6. Harvest the cells onto glass fiber filters with the aid of a cell harvester. Determine [^{3}H-methyl] thymidine uptake.
7. Calculate IL-5 concentration by comparison to rIL-5 standard curve. Using semilog or probit paper, plot standard IL-5 concentration on the *x*-axis vs. proliferation (in cpm) on the *y*-axis. Calculate the sample concentration by comparison to standard curve and multiplication by dilution factor.

Comments

1. A proliferation assay with TF-1 cells (ATCC Cat. No. CRL 2003) can be used as a bioassay for the measurement of human IL-5 (See Section C). This cell line, however, responds also to IL-3, IL-4, IL-6, and GM-CSF; thus, neutralization with appropriate monoclonal antibodies is advised to ascertain specificity.

F. *Interleukin-6*

Interleukin-6 (IL-6) is a highly pleiotropic cytokine synthesized by activated T (Th2) and B cells and a variety of non-lymphoid cells, including monocyte/macrophages, fibroblasts, endothelial cells, keratinocytes, and several tumor cells.[72] IL-6 plays a central role as a mediator of inflammatory and acute phase responses.[2,72] In addition, IL-6 exerts many other activities, such as induction of proliferation and differentiation of activated B cells, induction of polyclonal immunoglobulin secretion, differentiation of CTLs, and promotion of growth of hybridomas, plasmacytomas, and several other malignant cells, including Kaposi's sarcoma and multiple myeloma.[72,73] The high-affinity receptor for IL-6 is a heterodimer composed of an IL-6-binding subunit (CD126, IL-6Rα, 80 kDa) that interacts with a signal-transducing subunit (CD130, IL-6Rβ, gp130) that is shared among receptors for IL-6, leukemia-inhibitory factor (LIF), and oncostatin-M.[74] Soluble IL-6 receptors have been reported in the urine and serum of humans.[75]

Although IL-6 has many different activities, its ability to act as a "hybridoma growth factor," inducing the proliferation of a number of IL-6-dependent hybridomas, is the basis for a simple and sensitive assay.

1. *Hybridoma Growth Factor Assay*

A number of IL-6-dependent hybridomas have been reported. Commonly used indicator cells for the assay of IL-6 are the B9[76] and the 7TD1 hybridomas.[77] Although of murine origin, these indicator cell lines respond to both human and mouse IL-6.

Materials and reagents

- B9 or 7TD1 (ATCC Cat. No. CRL 1851) hybridomas

- Recombinant mouse or human IL-6 standard
- Culture medium: RPMI-1640 containing 10% heat-inactivated FCS, 2 m*M* L-glutamine, 10 m*M* HEPES, 100 U/ml penicillin, 100 μg/ml streptomycin, 50 μ*M* 2-mercaptoethanol, and 1 m*M* sodium pyruvate
- Washing buffer: PBS containing 1% FCS (filter-sterilized)
- [^{3}H-methyl] thymidine
- 96-well tissue culture plates (flat bottom)
- 15- and 50-ml centrifuge tubes
- Pasteur pipettes
- Refrigerated centrifuge (set at 4°C)
- CO_2 incubator (humidified, set at 37°C and 5% CO_2)
- Cell harvester (e.g., Skatron)
- Glass fiber filter mats (Skatron)
- Scintillation vials
- Scintillation cocktail (e.g., Econo-Safe, Research Products International)
- Scintillation counter

Protocol

(*Note*: All materials and reagents must be sterile and proper aseptic techniques must be used when handling the cells.)

1. Harvest the indicator cells, and wash twice with washing buffer and once with culture medium to remove any IL-6. Centrifuge at 200*g* for 10 min. Count and resuspend the cells to a density of 2×10^4 cells/ml in culture medium.
2. Dilute test samples and standards (0.1 to 100 U/ml) in culture medium. Include a negative control containing medium only. Add 100 μl per well (in triplicate).
3. Add 100 μl of the indicator cell suspension to each well (final: 2000 cells/well).
4. Incubate the plate for 72 hr at 37°C and 5% CO_2.
5. Add 20 μl/well of a 50-μCi/ml solution of [^{3}H-methyl] thymidine in culture medium (final concentration is 1 μCi/well) during the last 4 hr of incubation.
6. Harvest the cells onto glass fiber mats with the aid of a cell harvester. Determine [^{3}H-methyl] thymidine uptake by liquid scintillation counting.
7. Calculate the IL-6 concentration by comparison to rIL-6 standard curve. Using semilog or probit paper, plot standard IL-6 concentration on the *x*-axis vs. proliferation (in cpm) on the *y*-axis. Calculate the sample concentration by comparison to standard curve and multiplication by dilution factor.

2. Maintenance of B9 or 7TD1 cells

Materials and reagents

- B9 or 7TD1 (ATCC Cat. No. CRL 1851) hybridomas
- Recombinant mouse or human IL-6 standard
- Culture medium: RPMI-1640 containing 10% heat-inactivated FCS and supplemented with 2 m*M* L-glutamine, 10 m*M* HEPES, 100 U/ml penicillin, 100 μg/ml streptomycin, 50 μ*M* 2-mercaptoethanol, and 1 m*M* sodium pyruvate
- 25-cm^2 culture flasks
- 15- and 50-ml centrifuge tubes
- Pasteur pipettes
- Refrigerated centrifuge (set at 4°C)
- CO_2 incubator (humidified, set at 37°C and 5% CO_2)

Protocol

(*Note:* All materials and reagents must be sterile and proper aseptic techniques must be used when handling the cells.)

1. Seed cells at an initial density of 5×10^4 cells/ml in culture medium containing rIL-6 (50 to 100 U/ml).
2. Culture at 37°C and 5% CO_2 until cell density reaches 1×10^6 cells/ml (approximately 3 to 4 days). At this point, the cells should be subcultured.
3. For the proliferation assay, use cells in the log phase of growth (2 to 3 days).

Comments

1. B9 cells have been reported to respond to IL-4, albeit with much lower sensitivity compared to IL-6 (approx. 1000-fold). Potential interference with IL-4 can thus be avoided by performing the assay in the presence of anti-IL-4 antibodies (11B11, 10 μg/ml). B9 cells are available from Dr. Lucien Aarden, Central Laboratory of The Netherlands Red Cross Transfusion Service, Amsterdam, The Netherlands.

G. Interleukin-7

Interleukin-7 (IL-7) is a cytokine produced by bone marrow and thymic stromal cells.[78,79] IL-7 was originally described as a factor that induced proliferation and supported *in vitro* growth of B cell precursors.[78] In addition, IL-7 has been shown to be mitogenic for thymocytes and to co-stimulate with mitogens the proliferation of mature T cells.[80,81] IL-7 functions as a T cell growth factor in ConA blasts or T cell lines in the absence of IL-2 or IL-4.[80,81] The effects of IL-7 are mediated by binding to high-affinity IL-7 receptors, which are composed of an IL-7Rα-subunit (CD127), responsible for ligand binding, and the cytokine receptor common γ_c subunit (CD132), responsible for signal transduction.[28,82] The γ_c subunit is the IL-2R γ chain, which is shared among receptors for IL-2, IL-4, IL-7, IL-13, and IL-15.[11,27-29] Human and murine IL-7 do not exhibit species specificity and are active in either system.[83]

Initially, IL-7 was assayed using progenitor B cells derived from long-term Whitlock-Witte cultures[84]; however, this was both a labor-intensive and time-consuming assay. IL-7 has also been assayed based on its ability to co-stimulate the proliferation of murine thymocytes in the presence of ConA[81]; however, this assay is not specific for IL-7, as a number of other cytokines (such as IL-1, IL-2, IL-4, and IL-6) also stimulate thymocyte proliferation under these conditions. More recently, IL-7-dependent immature B lymphocytic cell lines, such as 2E8[85] and Ixn/2bx[83] have become available, making possible the assay of IL-7 through a simple proliferation assay.

1. 2E8 proliferation assay

This assay is based on the ability of IL-7 to stimulate the proliferation of IL-7-dependent immature B lymphocyte cell line 2E8.[85] These cells respond to both human and murine IL-7.

Materials and reagents

- 2E8 cells (ATCC Cat. No. TIB 239)
- Recombinant mouse or human IL-7 standard
- Culture medium: Iscove's modified DMEM plus 20% FCS, 50 μ*M* 2-mercaptoethanol, 100 U/ml penicillin, and 100 μg/ml streptomycin
- Washing buffer: PBS containing 1% FCS
- [^{3}H-methyl] thymidine
- 96-well tissue culture plates (flat bottom)
- 15- and 50-ml centrifuge tubes
- Pasteur pipettes
- Refrigerated centrifuge (set at 4°C)
- CO_2 incubator (humidified, set at 37°C and 5% CO_2)
- Cell harvester (e.g., Skatron)
- Glass fiber filter mats (Skatron)
- Scintillation vials
- Scintillation cocktail (e.g., Econo-Safe, Research Products International)
- Scintillation counter

Protocol

(*Note*: All materials and reagents must be sterile and proper aseptic techniques must be used when handling the cells.)

1. Harvest the indicator cells, and wash twice with washing buffer and once with culture medium. Count and resuspend the cells to a density of 1×10^5 cells/ml in culture medium.
2. Dilute test samples and standards (0.1 to 100 U/ml) in culture medium. Include a negative control containing medium only. Add 50 µl per well (in triplicate).
3. Add 50 µl of the indicator cell suspension to each well (final: 5000 cells/well).
4. Incubate the plate for 48 hr at 37°C and 5% CO_2.
5. Add 20 µl/well of a 50-µCi/ml solution of [^{3}H-methyl] thymidine in culture medium (final concentration is 1 µCi/well) during the last 4 hr of incubation.
6. Harvest the cells onto glass fiber mats with the aid of a cell harvester. Determine [^{3}H-methyl] thymidine uptake by liquid scintillation counting.
7. Calculate the IL-7 concentration by comparison to rIL-7 standard curve. Using semilog or probit paper, plot standard IL-7 concentration on the *x*-axis vs. proliferation (in cpm) on the *y*-axis. Calculate the sample concentration by comparison to standard curve and multiplication by dilution factor.

2. Maintenance of 2E8 cells

Materials and reagents

- 2E8 cells (ATCC Cat. No. TIB 239)
- Recombinant mouse or human IL-7 standard
- Culture medium: Iscove's modified DMEM plus 20% FCS, 50 µ*M* 2-mercaptoethanol, 100 U/ml penicillin, and 100 µg/ml streptomycin
- Recombinant IL-7 (mouse or human)
- 25-cm^2 tissue culture flasks
- 15- and 50-ml centrifuge tubes
- Pasteur pipettes
- Refrigerated centrifuge (set at 4°C)
- CO_2 incubator (humidified, set at 37°C and 5% CO_2)

Protocol

(*Note*: All materials and reagents must be sterile and proper aseptic techniques must be used when handling the cells.)

1. Seed cells at an initial density of 1×10^4 cells/ml in culture medium containing rIL-7 (~1 ng/ml).
2. Culture at 37°C and 5% CO_2 until cell density reaches 5×10^5 cells/ml. At this point, the cells should be subcultured.
3. For the proliferation assay, use cells in the log phase of growth (2 to 3 days).

H. Interleukin-9

1. M-07e proliferation assay

Interleukin-9 (IL-9, P40/TGFIII) is a cytokine produced by T lymphocytes.[86,87] IL-9 has growth factor activity on a variety of cells, including T cells, mast cells, and myeloid and erythroid precursor cells.[87,88] A bioassay for IL-9 is based on its ability to stimulate the proliferation of an IL-9-dependent megakaryocytic leukemia cell line (M-07e).[87] This cell line is dependent on either human GM-CSF or IL-3 for growth, and also responds to IL-2, IL-4, and IL-6. Thus, although useful to quantify levels of IL-9 in the absence of other cytokines, analysis of complex mixtures of cytokines is more complicated and requires the use of specific blocking antibodies. The reagents necessary for the IL-9 bioassay, including the indicator cell line, recombinant IL-9 standard, and neutralizing anti-IL-9 antibodies, are available to academic laboratories from Genetics Institute (Cambridge, MA). Other commercial sources of rIL-9 are also available. This assay detects both human and mouse IL-9.

Materials and reagents

- M-07e cell line
- Recombinant human IL-9 standard
- Culture medium: RPMI-1640 containing 10% heat-inactivated FCS, 2 m*M* L-glutamine, 10 m*M* HEPES, 100 U/ml penicillin, 100 μg/ml streptomycin, 50 μ*M* 2-mercaptoethanol, and 1 m*M* sodium pyruvate
- Washing buffer: PBS containing 1% FCS (filter-sterilized)
- [^{3}H-methyl] thymidine
- 96-well tissue culture plates (flat bottom)
- 15- and 50-ml centrifuge tubes
- Pasteur pipettes
- Refrigerated centrifuge (set at 4°C)
- CO_2 incubator (humidified, set at 37°C and 5% CO_2)
- Cell harvester (e.g., Skatron)
- Glass fiber filter mats (Skatron)
- Scintillation vials
- Scintillation cocktail (e.g., Econo-Safe, Research Products International)
- Scintillation counter

Protocol

(*Note*: All materials and reagents must be sterile and proper aseptic techniques must be used when handling the cells.)

1. Harvest the indicator cells, and wash twice with washing buffer and once with culture medium to remove any GM-CSF or IL-3 used in cell maintenance. Centrifuge at 200 × *g* for 10 min. Count and resuspend the cells to a density of 1×10^5 cells/ml in culture medium.
2. Dilute test samples and standards (0.1 to 100 U/ml) in culture medium. Include a negative control containing medium only. Add 100 μl per well (in triplicate).
3. Add 100 μl of the indicator cell suspension to each well (final: 10,000 cells/well).
4. Incubate the plate for 72 hr at 37°C and 5% CO_2.
5. Add 20 μl/well of a 50-μCi/ml solution of [^{3}H-methyl] thymidine in culture medium (final concentration is 1 μCi/well) during the last 4 hr of incubation.
6. Harvest the cells onto glass fiber mats with the aid of a cell harvester. Determine [^{3}H-methyl] thymidine uptake by liquid scintillation counting.
7. Calculate the IL-9 concentration by comparison to rIL-9 standard curve. Using semilog or probit paper, plot standard IL-9 concentration on the *x*-axis vs. proliferation (in cpm) on the *y*-axis. Calculate the sample concentration by comparison to standard curve and multiplication by dilution factor.

2. Maintenance of M-07e cells

Materials and reagents

- M-07e cells
- Recombinant human GM-CSF or IL-3 stock
- Culture medium: RPMI-1640 containing 10% heat-inactivated FCS and supplemented with 2 m*M* L-glutamine, 10 m*M* HEPES, 100 U/ml penicillin, 100 μg/ml streptomycin, 50 μM 2-mercaptoethanol, and 1 m*M* sodium pyruvate
- 25-cm^2 culture flasks
- 15- and 50-ml centrifuge tubes
- Pasteur pipettes
- Refrigerated centrifuge (set at 4°C)
- CO_2 incubator (humidified, set at 37°C and 5% CO_2)

Protocol

(*Note*: All materials and reagents must be sterile and proper aseptic techniques must be used when handling the cells.)

1. Seed cells at an initial density of 3×10^5 cells/ml in culture medium containing rGM-CSF (100 U/ml) or IL-3 (8 U/ml).
2. Culture at 37°C and 5% CO_2 for approximately 3 to 4 days. At this point, the cells should be subcultured.
3. For the proliferation assay, collect cells after the third or fourth day of culture.

Comments

1. M-07e cells respond to GM-CSF and IL-3; thus assays of samples containing mixtures of cytokines should be carried out in the presence of neutralizing monoclonal antibodies.

I. Interleukin-10

Interleukin-10 (IL-10) is a cytokine produced by a subset of T cells (Th2), certain B cells, EBV-transformed B cell lines, and activated monocytes.[89] Originally, IL-10 was described as a product of Th2 cells that inhibited the cytokine secretion by Th1 cells and was thus termed cytokine-synthesis inhibitory factor (CSIF).[90] However, many other activities have been found to be induced by IL-10, including enhanced proliferation of thymocytes in the presence of IL-2 and IL-4, increased proliferation of mast cells in the presence of IL-3 and IL-4, inhibition of production of inflammatory cytokines (TNFα, IL-1) and antigen-presentation function in macrophages, and induction of growth and differentiation in activated human B cells.[89] An Epstein-Barr virus (EBV)-encoded protein (BCRF1) possesses extensive similarity with IL-10 and exhibits some, but not all, functions associated with IL-10, including cytokine synthesis inhibitory activity.[91]

The original assay for IL-10 was based on its ability to inhibit interferon-γ production by Th1 cell clones or mitogen-stimulated spleen cells.[90] More recently, a simple proliferation assay has been described based on the ability of IL-10 to enhance the proliferation of a mast cell line (MC/9)[41] in the presence of IL-4.[92] Both of these assays are described below. The indicator cells, murine Th1 clones or MC/9 cells, are responsive to both human and mouse IL-10.

1. Cytokine synthesis inhibition assay

In this assay, Th1 cells are first stimulated by antigen plus antigen-presenting cells in the presence of IL-10 standards or samples, followed by measurement of the amount of IFNγ contained in the supernatant after a 24- hour incubation. The presence of IL-10 causes a dose-dependent decrease in IFNγ secretion.

Materials and reagents

- Th1 cell clone (e.g., LB2-1; ATCC Cat. No. CRL 8629)

- Recombinant IL-10 standard (human or mouse)
- Mitomycin C-treated spleen cell suspension (from a strain syngeneic with Th1 cells; C57Bl/6 for LB2-1)
- Antigen (chicken red blood cells for LB2-1)
- Recombinant IL-2 (human or mouse)
- Culture medium: RPMI-1640 containing 10% heat-inactivated FCS and supplemented with 2 m*M* L-glutamine, 10 m*M* HEPES, 100 U/ml penicillin, 100 μg/ml streptomycin, 50 μ*M* 2-mercaptoethanol, and 1 m*M* sodium pyruvate
- Washing buffer: PBS containing 1% FCS (filter-sterilized)
- 96-well tissue culture plates (flat bottom)
- 15- and 50-ml centrifuge tubes
- Pasteur pipettes
- Refrigerated centrifuge (set at 4°C)
- CO_2 incubator (humidified, set at 37°C and 5% CO_2)
- Additional materials for assay of IFNγ (bioassay [see Section R] or ELISA)

Protocol

(*Note:* All materials and reagents must be sterile and proper aseptic techniques must be used when handling the cells.)

1. Prepare a splenic cell suspension, wash once with washing buffer, and resuspend in culture medium to a cell density of 1×10^7 cells/ml. Incubate the cells with mitomycin C at a final concentration of 50 μg/ml for 30 min at 37°C. Wash the cells 4× with 20 ml ice-cold washing buffer, centrifuging at 200*g* for 10 min. Assess viability and resuspend the cells in culture medium to 2×10^7 cells/ml. Alternatively, cells can be irradiated at 2500 rad.
2. Harvest "rested" Th1 cells (Th1 cells should be used no earlier than 7 days after the last stimulation). Wash once with washing buffer and once with culture medium. Count and resuspend to a density of 2×10^6 cells/ml in culture medium containing rIL-2 (4 ng/ml) and the appropriate concentration of antigen (0.04% chicken red blood cells for LB2-1 cells).
3. Dilute samples and standards in culture medium. Add 50 μl per well. Assay each dilution in triplicate.
4. Mix equal volumes of the spleen cell and Th1 cell suspensions (Steps 1 and 2) and add 50 μl per well. Incubate for 24 hr at 37°C and 5% CO_2.
5. Collect ~75 μl of supernatant from each well, making sure not to get any cells from the bottom.
6. Assay supernatants for IFNγ (see Section N in this chapter).
7. Calculate IL-10 concentration by reference to an rIL-10 standard curve. Using semilog paper, plot standard IL-10 concentration on the *x*-axis vs. IFNγ production on the *y*-axis. Calculate sample concentration by comparison to standard curve and multiplication by dilution factor.

Comments

1. For a basic protocol for the maintenance of the T cell clones, refer to Section A.3 in this chapter. Alternatively, this assay can be performed with ConA-stimulated splenic cells instead of Th1 clones.
2. The presence of IL-2 or IL-4 in the samples may affect this assay due to an increase of IFNγ production, whereas the presence of transforming growth factor-β (TGF-β) may decrease it. If samples are suspected of containing these cytokines, perform the assay in the presence of neutralizing antibodies against these cytokines.

2. MC/9 proliferation assay

This assay is based on the ability of IL-10 to enhance the proliferation of MC/9 cells, a mast cell line, in the presence of rIL-4.

Materials and reagents

- MC/9 cells (ATCC Cat. No. CRL 8306)
- Recombinant mouse or human IL-10 standard
- Recombinant mouse IL-4
- Culture medium: RPMI-1640 containing 10% heat-inactivated FCS and supplemented with 2 m*M* L-glutamine, 10 m*M* HEPES, 100 U/ml penicillin, 100 μg/ml streptomycin, 50 μ*M* 2-mercaptoethanol, and 1 m*M* sodium pyruvate
- Washing buffer: PBS containing 1% FCS
- [^{3}H-methyl] thymidine
- 96-well tissue culture plates (flat bottom)
- 15- and 50-ml centrifuge tubes
- Pasteur pipettes
- Refrigerated centrifuge (set at 4°C)
- CO_2 incubator (humidified, set at 37°C and 5% CO_2)
- Cell harvester (e.g., Skatron)
- Glass fiber filter mats (Skatron)
- Scintillation vials
- Scintillation cocktail (e.g., Econo-Safe, Research Products International)
- Scintillation counter

Protocol

(*Note*: All materials and reagents must be sterile and proper aseptic techniques must be used when handling the cells.)

1. Harvest the indicator cells, and wash twice with washing buffer and once with culture medium. Count and resuspend the cells to a density of 5×10^4 cells/ml in culture medium containing 400 pg/ml of rIL-4.

Background proliferation can be reduced by harvesting the MC/9 cells on the day before the assay and culturing them overnight (after washing) in culture medium without rIL-3 or the ConA-spleen cell conditioned medium (see protocol for maintenance of MC/9 cells below).

2. Dilute test samples and standards (0.1 to 100 U/ml) in complete medium. Include a negative control containing medium only. Add 100 μl per well (in triplicate).
3. Add 100 μl of the indicator cell suspension to each well (final: 5000 cells/well).
4. Incubate the plate for 72 hr at 37°C and 5% CO_2.
5. Add 20 μl/well of a 50-μCi/ml solution of [^{3}H-methyl] thymidine in culture medium (final concentration is 1 μCi/well) during the last 4 hr of incubation.
6. Harvest the cells onto glass fiber filters with the aid of a cell harvester. Determine [^{3}H-methyl] thymidine uptake by liquid scintillation counting.
7. Calculate the IL-10 concentration by comparison to rIL-10 standard curve. Using semilog or probit paper, plot standard IL-10 concentration on the *x*-axis vs. proliferation (in cpm) on the *y*-axis. Calculate the sample concentration by comparison to standard curve and multiplication by dilution factor.

3. Maintenance of MC/9 cells

Materials and reagents

- MC/9 cells (ATCC Cat. No. CRL 8306)
- Recombinant mouse IL-3 or ConA-activated splenic cell conditioned medium
- Culture medium: RPMI-1640 containing 10% heat-inactivated FCS and supplemented with 2 m*M* L-glutamine, 10 m*M* HEPES, 100 U/ml penicillin, 100 μg/ml streptomycin, 50 μ*M* 2-mercaptoethanol, and 1 m*M* sodium pyruvate
- 25-cm^2 tissue culture flasks
- 15- and 50-ml centrifuge tubes
- Pasteur pipettes
- Refrigerated centrifuge (set at 4°C)
- CO_2 incubator (humidified, set at 37°C and 5% CO_2)

Protocol

(*Note*: All materials and reagents must be sterile and proper aseptic techniques must be used when handling the cells.)

1. Seed cells at an initial density of 5 × 10^4 cells/ml in culture medium containing rIL-3 or 5% ConA-activated splenic cell-conditioned medium (a source of growth factors). To prepare the ConA-supernatant,

culture murine spleen cells at a final cell density of 1 × 10^7 cells/ml in culture medium containing ConA (5 μg/ml) for 24 hr at 37°C and 5% CO_2. Harvest by centrifugation, filter, and store at –20°C.

2. Culture at 37°C and 5% CO_2 for 3 days. At this point, the cells should be subcultured.
3. For the proliferation assay, use cells in the log phase of growth (2 to 3 days).

Comments

1. IL-3 and IL-4 stimulate proliferation of mast cells and synergize with IL-10. Their presence in samples may affect the results. MC/9 cells also respond to murine and human stem cell factor (SCF or *c-kit* ligand).

J. Interleukin-11

Interleukin-11 (IL-11) is a cytokine originally described as a product of a bone marrow stromal cell line that induced proliferation of an IL-6-dependent plasmacytoma cell line (T1165).[93] In addition to this activity, IL-11 has been demonstrated to have a growth-promoting effect on some hemopoietic precursor cells (including megakaryocytic and erythroid lineages) and lymphoid cells.[93] IL-11 appears to share some functions in common with IL-6, such as acting as an adipogenesis-inhibiting factor and inducing synthesis of acute-phase proteins by liver cells.[94] The IL-11 receptor shares the gp130 signal-transducing subunit with the IL-6R.[95]

1. T10 proliferation assay

A bioassay for IL-11 is based on its ability to stimulate the proliferation of murine T10 cells, a subline derived from the parental T1165 cell line.[96] T10 cells are maintained in the presence of human rIL-11 and respond to both human and mouse IL-11. These cells, however, retain their ability to proliferate in response to IL-6. Specific blocking antibodies can be used to distinguish the activities of IL-6 and IL-11. The reagents for this assay, including the indicator cell line, recombinant IL-11 standard, and neutralizing anti-IL-11 antibodies, are available to academic laboratories from Genetics Institute (Cambridge, MA). Other commercial sources of rIL-11 are also available.

Materials and reagents

- T10 cell line
- Recombinant human IL-11 standard
- Culture medium: RPMI-1640 containing 10% heat-inactivated FCS, 2 m*M* L-glutamine, 10 m*M* HEPES, 100 U/ml penicillin, 100 μg/ml streptomycin, 50 μ*M* 2-mercaptoethanol, and 1 m*M* sodium pyruvate

- Washing buffer: PBS containing 1% FCS (filter-sterilized)
- [^{3}H-methyl] thymidine
- 96-well tissue culture plates (flat bottom)
- 15- and 50-ml centrifuge tubes
- Pasteur pipettes
- Refrigerated centrifuge (set at 4°C)
- CO_2 incubator (humidified, set at 37°C and 5% CO_2)
- Cell harvester (e.g., Skatron)
- Glass fiber filter mats (Skatron)
- Scintillation vials
- Scintillation cocktail (e.g., Econo-Safe, Research Products International)
- Scintillation counter

Protocol

(*Note*: All materials and reagents must be sterile and proper aseptic techniques must be used when handling the cells.)

1. Harvest the indicator cells, and wash twice with washing buffer and once with culture medium to remove any rIL-11 used in cell maintenance. Centrifuge at 200*g* for 10 min. Count and resuspend the cells to a density of 0.75×10^5 cells/ml in culture medium.
2. Dilute test samples and standards (0.1 to 100 U/ml) in culture medium. Include a negative control containing medium only. Add 100 μl per well (in triplicate).
3. Add 100 μl of the indicator cell suspension to each well (final: 7500 cells/well).
4. Incubate the plate for 72 hr at 37°C and 5% CO_2.
5. Add 20 μl/well of a 50-μCi/ml solution of [^{3}H-methyl] thymidine in culture medium (final concentration is 1 μCi/well) during the last 4 hr of incubation.
6. Harvest the cells onto glass fiber mats with the aid of a cell harvester. Determine [^{3}H-methyl] thymidine uptake by liquid scintillation counting.
7. Calculate the IL-11 concentration by comparison to rIL-11 standard curve. Using semilog or probit paper, plot standard IL-11 concentration on the *x*-axis vs. proliferation (in cpm) on the *y*-axis. Calculate sample concentration by comparison to standard curve and multiplication by dilution factor.

2. Maintenance of T10 cells

Materials and reagents

- T10 cells
- Recombinant human IL-11 stock

- Culture medium: RPMI-1640 containing 10% heat-inactivated FCS and supplemented with 2 m*M* L-glutamine, 10 m*M* HEPES, 100 U/ml penicillin, 100 μg/ml streptomycin, 50 μ*M* 2-mercaptoethanol, and 1 m*M* sodium pyruvate
- 25-cm^2 culture flasks
- 15- and 50-ml centrifuge tubes
- Pasteur pipettes
- Refrigerated centrifuge (set at 4°C)
- CO_2 incubator (humidified, set at 37°C and 5% CO_2)

Protocol

(*Note*: All materials and reagents must be sterile and proper aseptic techniques must be used when handling the cells.)

1. Seed cells at an initial density of 5×10^5 cells/ml in culture medium containing rIL-11 (20 U/ml).
2. Culture at 37°C and 5% CO_2 for approximately 3 to 4 days. At this point, the cells should be subcultured.
3. For the proliferation assay, collect cells after the third or fourth day of culture.

Comments

1. T10 cells respond to IL-11 and IL-6; thus, assay of samples containing contaminating IL-6 should be performed in the presence of the appropriate blocking anti-IL-6 and anti-IL-11 antibodies.

K. *Interleukin-12*

Interleukin-12 (IL-12) is a heterodimeric cytokine produced by a variety of cells, including macrophages, B cells, and keratinocytes, that was originally described by its ability to stimulate cytotoxicity of NK cells and maturation of CTLs.[97,98] IL-12 has multiple effects on T cells and NK cells, inducing the secretion of IFNγ from resting and activated cells and acting as a co-stimulant for the proliferation of T cells in the presence of mitogens.[97,99] Partly because of its ability to induce IFNγ synthesis, IL-12 has been shown to promote the development of Th1 responses and to inhibit that of Th2.[100]

Bioassays for IL-12 were originally based on its ability to stimulate the production of IFNγ from unstimulated peripheral blood mononuclear cells (PBMC), or to stimulate the proliferation of human PHA-stimulated T cell blasts.[97,99] This latter assay, however, lacks specificity for IL-12, making necessary the inclusion of neutralizing anti-IL-12 antibodies (when assaying samples potentially containing other cytokines in addition to IL-12) to confirm that the observed proliferation is due to IL-12. A modification of the PHA-blast proliferation assay has been reported,[101] in which samples are first incubated in wells containing immobilized anti-IL-12 antibodies and then the captured IL-12 is detected by adding PHA-blasts and measuring proliferation.

1. IFNγ induction assay for IL-12

In this assay, human PBMC are cultured in the presence of IL-12-containing samples, followed by collection of the supernatants which are later assayed for IFNγ.

Materials and reagents

- Suspension of human peripheral blood mononuclear cells (PBMC)
- Histopaque-1077 (Sigma Cat. No. H-8889)
- Blood collection tubes (heparinized)
- Recombinant (human) IL-12 standard
- Culture medium: RPMI-1640 containing 10% heat-inactivated FCS and supplemented with 2 m*M* L-glutamine, 10 m*M* HEPES, 100 U/ml penicillin, 100 μg/ml streptomycin, 50 μ*M* 2-mercaptoethanol, and 1 m*M* sodium pyruvate
- Washing buffer: PBS containing 1% FCS (filter-sterilized)
- Sterile PBS
- 100 × 15-mm Petri dishes
- 96-well tissue culture plates (flat bottom)
- 15- and 50-ml centrifuge tubes
- Pasteur pipettes
- Refrigerated centrifuge (set at 4°C)
- CO_2 incubator (humidified, set at 37°C and 5% CO_2)
- Additional materials for assay of IFNγ (bioassay [see Section R] or ELISA)

Protocol

(*Note*: All materials and reagents must be sterile and proper aseptic techniques must be used when handling the cells.)

1. Collect blood (heparinized) from healthy human donors and isolate PBMC by density gradient centrifugation using Histopaque-1077 (see Chapter 1). Wash cells in sterile PBS, count, and resuspend in culture medium at 5×10^6 cells/ml and deplete adherent cells by incubation on plastic Petri dishes for 1 hr at 37°C. Repeat adherence procedure once more.
2. Resuspend PBMC in culture medium to a density of 4×10^6 cells/ml. Add 100 μl per well.
3. Dilute samples and standards (20 to 2000 pg/ml) with culture medium. Test each dilution in triplicate, including a negative control containing medium only. Add 100 μl per well.
4. Incubate at 37°C and 5% CO_2 for 12 hr.

5. Remove approximately 100 μl of supernatant, making sure not to take any cells from the bottom of the plate.
6. Assay supernatants for human IFNγ (see IFNγ assay later in this chapter).
7. Calculate the IL-12 concentration. Plot standard IL-12 concentration on the *x*-axis vs. IFNγ production on the *y*-axis. Calculate the sample concentration by comparison to standard curve and multiplication by dilution factor.

2. Lymphoblast proliferation assay for IL-12

This assay is based on the ability of IL-12 to induce proliferation of PHA-activated human T cell blasts. As other cytokines, such as IL-2 and IL-4 could also score in this assay, neutralization of IL-12 with monoclonal antibodies is recommended in order to confirm that the response is due to IL-12. This assay can detect either human or murine IL-12.

Materials and reagents

- Suspension of PBMC
- Histopaque-1077 (Sigma Cat. No. H-8889)
- Blood collection tubes (heparinized)
- Recombinant (human or mouse) IL-12 standard
- Phytohemagglutinin-P (PHA; Sigma Cat. No. L-9132)
- Culture medium: RPMI-1640 containing 10% heat-inactivated FCS and supplemented with 2 m*M* L-glutamine, 10 m*M* HEPES, 100 U/ml penicillin, 100 μg/ml streptomycin, 50 μ*M* 2-mercaptoethanol, and 1 m*M* sodium pyruvate
- Washing buffer: PBS containing 1% FCS (filter-sterilized)
- Sterile PBS
- [^{3}H-methyl] thymidine
- 75-cm^2 tissue culture flasks
- 96-well tissue culture plates (flat bottom)
- 15- and 50-ml centrifuge tubes
- Pasteur pipettes
- Refrigerated centrifuge (set at 4°C)
- CO_2 incubator (humidified, set at 37°C and 5% CO_2)
- Cell harvester (e.g., Skatron)
- Glass fiber filter mats (Skatron)
- Scintillation vials
- Scintillation cocktail (e.g., Econo-Safe, Research Products International)
- Scintillation counter

Protocol

(*Note*: All materials and reagents must be sterile and proper aseptic techniques must be used when handling the cells.)

1. Prepare PBMC by density gradient centrifugation, as in previous section. Wash three times with sterile PBS, assess viability, and resuspend in culture medium to a density of 5×10^5 cells/ml.
2. Add enough PHA from a 5-mg/ml stock solution in culture medium to the cell suspension to obtain a final PHA concentration of 5 µg/ml. Culture for 72 hr at 37°C and 5% CO_2 using 75-cm^2 tissue culture flasks.
3. Split cells 1:2 with culture medium. Add rIL-2 (human) to a final concentration of 50 U/ml. Incubate for an additional 24 hr.
4. Harvest the cells into 50-ml centrifuge tubes, and wash twice with ice-cold washing buffer and once with culture medium to remove the rIL-2.
5. Count the cells and resuspend the lymphoblasts in culture medium to a cell density of 4×10^5 cells/ml. Add 50 µl per well.
6. Dilute samples and standards (20 to 2000 pg/ml) with culture medium. Add 50 µl per well. Include negative controls containing medium alone. Assay each dilution in triplicate.
7. Incubate for 24 hr at 37°C and 5% CO_2.
8. Add 20 µl/well of a 50-µCi/ml solution of [^{3}H-methyl] thymidine in culture medium (final concentration is 1 µCi/well) during the last 4 to 6 hr of incubation.
9. Harvest the cells onto glass fiber mats with the aid of a cell harvester. Determine [^{3}H-methyl] thymidine uptake by liquid scintillation counting.
10. Calculate the IL-12 concentration by comparison to rIL-12 standard curve. Using semilog or probit paper, plot standard IL-12 concentration on the *x*-axis vs. proliferation (in cpm) on the *y*-axis. Calculate the sample concentration by comparison to standard curve and multiplication by dilution factor.

Comments

1. This assay detects both human and mouse IL-12. Because the indicator cells are of human origin, the possible interference by murine IL-2 or IL-4 (which are not active on human cells) is avoided. This, however, is not the case with human samples.

L. *Interleukin-13*

Interleukin-13 (IL-13) is a cytokine produced primarily by subsets of T cells (Th2 cells).[102] IL-13 has moderate sequence homology (25 to 30%) to IL-4, and shares with it a number of biological activities in the human, including upregulation of B cell class II MHC and CD23 molecule expression, B cell proliferation and secretion of IgE, and inhibition of production of inflammatory cytokines by macrophages.[102-105] In the mouse, however, IL-13 appears to modulate mostly the monocytic lineage.[106] Moreover, the IL-13 receptor shares a common signal-transducing subunit (γ_c chain) with receptors for IL-2, IL-4, IL-7, and IL-15.[11,27-29]

The bioassays for IL-13 is based on its ability to induce the proliferation of the B9 hybridoma.[107] This is basically the same proliferation assay used for the assay of IL-6 (see Section F in this chapter). B9 cells also respond to IL-6 and, to a lesser extent, IL-4. Both human and mouse IL-13 are detected by this assay. IL-13 can also be assayed using TF-1 human erythroleukemia cells (see Section C, this chapter).

1. B9 proliferation assay for IL-13

Materials and reagents

- B9 hybridoma
- Recombinant mouse or human IL-13 standard
- Culture medium: RPMI-1640 containing 10% heat-inactivated FCS and supplemented with 2 m*M* L-glutamine, 10 m*M* HEPES, 100 U/ml penicillin, 100 μg/ml streptomycin, 50 μ*M* 2-mercaptoethanol, and 1 m*M* sodium pyruvate
- Washing buffer: PBS containing 1% FCS (filter-sterilized)
- [^{3}H-methyl] thymidine
- 96-well tissue culture plates (flat bottom)
- 15- and 50-ml centrifuge tubes
- Pasteur pipettes
- Refrigerated centrifuge (set at 4°C)
- CO_2 incubator (humidified, set at 37°C and 5% CO_2)
- Cell harvester (e.g., Skatron)
- Glass fiber filter mats (Skatron)
- Scintillation vials
- Scintillation cocktail (e.g., Econo-Safe, Research Products International)
- Scintillation counter

Protocol

(*Note*: All materials and reagents must be sterile and proper aseptic techniques must be used when handling the cells.)

1. Harvest the indicator cells, and wash twice with washing buffer and once with culture medium to remove any rIL-6. Count and resuspend the cells to a density of 1 × 10^5 cells/ml in culture medium.

2. Dilute test samples and standards (20 to 2000 pg/ml) in culture medium. Include a negative control containing medium only. Add 50 μl per well (in triplicate).
3. Add 50 μl of the indicator cell suspension to each well (final: 5000 cells/well).
4. Incubate the plate for 48 to 72 hr at 37°C and 5% CO_2.
5. Add 20 μl/well of a 50-μCi/ml solution of [^{3}H-methyl] thymidine in culture medium (final concentration is 1 μCi/well) during the last 4 to 6 hr of incubation.
6. Harvest the cells onto glass fiber mats with the aid of a cell harvester. Determine [^{3}H-methyl] thymidine uptake by liquid scintillation counting.
7. Calculate the IL-13 concentration by comparison to rIL-13 standard curve. Using semilog or probit paper, plot standard IL-13 concentration on the *x*-axis vs. proliferation (in cpm) on the *y*-axis. Calculate the sample concentration by comparison to standard curve and multiplication by dilution factor.

Comments

1. For the maintenance of B9 cells, refer to Section F in this chapter.
2. B9 cells proliferate also in response to IL-6 and IL-4. When assaying murine samples, include neutralizing anti-IL-6 and anti-IL-4 antibodies if the presence of these cytokines is suspected. When assaying human samples, only anti-human IL-6 antibodies are required, as human IL-4 is not active on murine cells.
3. As with other cytokine assays, confirmation of IL-13 activity by inhibition with anti-IL-13 antibodies is recommended.

M. Interleukin-15

Interleukin-15 (IL-15) is a cytokine produced by a variety of cells, including adherent PBMC, epithelial, and fibroblast cell lines.[11] IL-15 shares many activities with IL-2, including the proliferation of activated human and mouse T cells and generation of LAK cells.[11,107] The IL-15 receptor appears to share with the IL-2R, both the β- and γ_c-subunits, since antibodies directed against the IL-2Rβ subunit block both IL-2 and IL-15 activity.[11]

The bioassay for IL-15 is based on its ability to stimulate the proliferation of CTLL-2 cells.[11] Inasmuch as IL-2 also stimulates the proliferation of this cell line, identification of IL-15 requires its neutralization with anti-IL-15 or anti-IL-2Rβ chain monoclonal antibodies, but not by anti-IL-2 or IL-2Rα antibodies.

1. CTLL-2 proliferation assay for IL-15

Materials and reagents

- CTLL-2 cells (ATCC Cat. No. TIB 214)

- Recombinant IL-15 standard
- Rat monoclonal anti-mouse IL-4 (11B11) (ATCC Cat. No. HB 188)
- Rat monoclonal anti-mouse IL-2 (S4B6) (ATCC Cat. No. HB 8794)
- Rat monoclonal anti-mouse IL-2Rβ (CD122) (BD Pharmingen, Cat. No. 01921D)
- Culture medium: RPMI-1640 containing 10% heat-inactivated FCS and supplemented with 2 m*M* L-glutamine, 10 m*M* HEPES, 100 U/ml penicillin, 100 μg/ml streptomycin, 50 μ*M* 2-mercaptoethanol, and 1 m*M* sodium pyruvate
- Washing buffer: PBS containing 1% FCS (filter-sterilized)
- [^{3}H-methyl] thymidine
- 96-well tissue culture plates (flat bottom)
- 15- and 50-ml centrifuge tubes
- Pasteur pipettes
- Refrigerated centrifuge (set at 4°C)
- CO_2 incubator (humidified, set at 37°C and 5% CO_2)
- Cell harvester (e.g., Skatron)
- Glass fiber filter mats (Skatron)
- Scintillation vials
- Scintillation cocktail (e.g., Econo-Safe, Research Products International)
- Scintillation counter

Protocol

(*Note*: All materials and reagents must be sterile and proper aseptic techniques must be used when handling the cells.)

1. Harvest the CTLL-2 cells (see Section B in this chapter), and wash twice with cold washing buffer and once with complete medium to remove any IL-2. Count and resuspend the cells in culture medium to 2.5×10^5 cells/ml.
2. Dilute samples and standards (1 to 100 ng/ml) in culture medium. Assay each dilution in triplicate. Include a negative control containing medium alone.
3. Add 20 to 50 μl of sample or recombinant IL-15 standard per well.
4. In the case of assays involving murine samples, the assay can be made specific for IL-15 by including neutralizing anti-IL-2 and anti-IL-4 antibodies (final concentration 10 μg/ml). In the case of human samples, only anti-human IL-2 antibodies need to be used (human IL-4 is not active in murine systems). Preincubate samples and antibodies for 30 min at room temperature.
5. Add sufficient culture medium to bring the volume of each well to 80 μl.
6. Add 20 μl of the indicator cell suspension to each well (5000 cells/well). The final volume is 100 μl. Incubate for 24 hr at 37°C in a 5% CO_2 atmosphere.

7. Add 20 μl/well of a 50-μCi/ml solution of [^{3}H-methyl] thymidine in culture medium (final concentration is 1 μCi/well) during the last 4 to 6 hr of incubation.
8. Harvest the cells onto glass fiber mats with the aid of a cell harvester. Determine [^{3}H-methyl] thymidine uptake by liquid scintillation counting.
9. Calculate the IL-15 concentration by comparison to rIL-15 standard curve. Using semilog or probit paper, plot standard IL-15 concentration on the x-axis vs. proliferation (in cpm) on the y-axis. Calculate the sample concentration by comparison to standard curve and multiplication by dilution factor.

Comments

1. Refer to Section B in this chapter for the maintenance of CTLL-2 cells.
2. Proliferation of CTLL-2 cells to IL-15 is blocked by antibodies against the IL-2Rβ subunit (CD122), but not against the IL-2R α-chain (CD25).
3. This assay detects both human and mouse IL-15.

N. Interleukin-16

Interleukin-16 (IL-16) is a cytokine that was first described based on its chemotactic properties for lymphocytes, thus its original name of Lymphocyte Chemoattractant Factor.[108] However, IL-16 is not a member of the chemokine family. The CD4 molecule acts as a receptor for IL-16, as demonstrated by blocking experiments with anti-CD4 antibodies or soluble CD4 molecules, and by transfection of murine T cells with human CD4. In addition to acting as a chemoattractant for $CD4^+$ T cells, IL-16 appears to regulate the activation of T cells, inducing the expression of the IL-2Rα subunit (CD25) and their progression from G_0 to G_1 in the cell cycle.[109] IL-16 also displays immunosuppressive effects on MLR and TCR/CD3-mediated activation, possibly due to interference with the normal action of CD4.[110] Functional assays for IL-16 are based on its chemotactic properties for $CD4^+$ T cells and other cell types such as monocytes or eosinophils. In addition, functional assays of IL-16 based on its ability to induce the expression of CD25 by primary human T cells or the entry of T cell lines into cycle have also been reported.[111] In all cases, neutralization of IL-16 activity with appropriate monoclonal antibodies is required for confirmation.

1. Chemotaxis of $CD4^+$ T cells

The activity of IL-16 can be assayed by measuring its stimulatory effects on the chemotaxis of isolated peripheral blood T cells or T cell lines, and demonstration of its inhibition by blocking anti-IL-16 antibodies. The basic assay for the measurement of chemotaxis is described in the chapter on chemokines (Chapter 7), and the isolation of T cells is described in Chapter 1.

2. *Induction of CD25 expression*

Materials and reagents

- T cells, isolated from peripheral blood (Chapter 1) or cultured $CD4^+$ T cell line, such as HUT 78 (ATCC Cat. No. TIB161)
- Recombinant IL-16 standard (human)
- Culture medium: RPMI-1640 containing 10% heat-inactivated FCS and supplemented with 2 m*M* L-glutamine, 10 m*M* HEPES, 100 U/ml penicillin, 100 μg/ml streptomycin, 50 μ*M* 2-mercaptoethanol, and 1 m*M* sodium pyruvate
- Washing buffer: PBS containing 1% FCS (filter-sterilized)
- Staining buffer: PBS containing 1% FCS and 10 m*M* sodium azide (kept ice cold)
- Fluorochrome-coupled monoclonal anti-human CD25 antibody and isotype-matched control (e.g., BD Pharmingen)
- 24-well tissue culture plates (flat bottom)
- 15- and 50-ml centrifuge tubes
- Pasteur pipettes
- Refrigerated centrifuge (set at 4°C)
- CO_2 incubator (humidified, set at 37°C and 5% CO_2)
- Flow cytometer

Protocol

(*Note*: All materials and reagents must be sterile and proper aseptic and biosafety techniques must be used when handling the cells.)

1. Prepare peripheral blood T cells or harvest indicator HUT 78 cells, wash twice with washing buffer and once with culture medium. Count and resuspend the cells to a density of 2×10^6 cells/ml in culture medium. Add 2 ml of the T cell suspension per well.
2. Dilute test samples and standards (enough to obtain a final concentration of 0.01 to 10 n*M*) in culture medium. Include a negative control (medium only) and a positive control containing a mitogen (e.g., ConA or PHA at 1 to 5 μg/ml). Add to wells.
3. Incubate the plate for 48 hr at 37°C and 5% CO_2.
4. After the incubation, transfer the contents of each well into individual tubes. Centrifuge at 300*g* for 10 min and remove the supernatant.
5. Wash the cells once with ice-cold staining buffer. Remove the supernatant and resuspend the cell pellets in 100 μl of staining buffer. Add 5 μl of labeled anti-CD25 antibody or isotype-matched control, diluted according to the manufacturer's recommendations.

6. Incubate the tubes on ice for 45 min. Avoid exposing the tubes to direct light.
7. Wash the cells twice with staining buffer (~3 ml each). After the final wash, resuspend the cells in 1 ml staining buffer if they are to be analyzed immediately. Alternatively, the cells can be fixed using PBS/10% formalin and analyzed at a later time.
8. Analyze in the flow cytometer. Measure increase in cell fluorescence in comparison to negative control and isotype-matched control antibody.

3. Proliferation of CD4+ T cell lines

Materials and reagents

- HUT 78 CD4+ T cell line (ATCC Cat. No. TIB161)
- Recombinant IL-16 standard
- Monoclonal anti-human IL-16 (BD Pharmingen, Cat. No. 20980D)
- Culture medium: RPMI-1640 containing 10% heat-inactivated FCS and supplemented with 2 m*M* L-glutamine, 10 m*M* HEPES, 100 U/ml penicillin, 100 µg/ml streptomycin, 50 µ*M* 2-mercaptoethanol, and 1 m*M* sodium pyruvate
- Washing buffer: PBS containing 1% FCS (filter-sterilized)
- [^{3}H-methyl] thymidine
- 96-well tissue culture plates (flat bottom)
- 15- and 50-ml centrifuge tubes
- Pasteur pipettes
- Refrigerated centrifuge (set at 4°C)
- CO_2 incubator (humidified, set at 37°C and 5% CO_2)
- Cell harvester (e.g., Skatron)
- Glass fiber filter mats (Skatron)
- Scintillation vials
- Scintillation cocktail (e.g., Econo-Safe, Research Products International)
- Scintillation counter

Protocol

(*Note*: All materials and reagents must be sterile and proper aseptic techniques must be used when handling the cells.)

1. Harvest the HUT 78 cells, and wash twice with cold washing buffer and once with complete medium. Count and resuspend the cells in culture medium to 0.5–1 × 10^6 cells/ml. Add 100 µl of the cell suspension per well in a 96-well plate.
2. Dilute samples and standards (0.01 to 10 n*M*) in culture medium. Add 100 µl of each dilution per well. Assay in triplicate. Include a negative control containing medium alone.

3. Incubate for 24 hr at 37°C in a 5% CO_2 atmosphere.
4. Add 20 μl/well of a 50-μCi/ml solution of [^{3}H-methyl] thymidine in culture medium (final concentration is 1 μCi/well) during the last 4 to 6 hr of incubation.
5. Harvest the cells onto glass fiber mats with the aid of a cell harvester. Determine [^{3}H-methyl] thymidine uptake by liquid scintillation counting.
6. Calculate the IL-16 concentration by comparison to rIL-16 standard curve. Using semilog or probit paper, plot standard IL-16 concentration on the *x*-axis vs. proliferation (in cpm) on the *y*-axis. Calculate the sample concentration by comparison to standard curve and multiplication by dilution factor.

Comments

1. Samples containing mixtures of cytokines should be retested in the presence of blocking anti-IL-16 antibodies to confirm that the proliferation is due to IL-16.

O. Interleukin-17

Interleukin-17 (IL-17) is a homodimeric cytokine produced by activated memory CD4$^+$ T cells that induces the production of cytokines such as IL-6, IL-8, and GM-CSF, as well as prostaglandin E2, from epithelial, endothelial, and fibroblastic cells.[112,113] IL-17 has a viral counterpart, HSV13 (vIL-17), a secretory glycoprotein produced by *Herpesvirus saimiri*, which displays similar biological activities.[112,113] Fibroblasts cultured in the presence of IL-17 sustain the proliferation of CD34$^+$ hemopoietic precursors and their preferential maturation into neutrophils.[112] These activities have suggested that IL-17 may function as an early initiator of T cell-dependent inflammatory reactions, as well as a linkage between the immune system and hemopoiesis. The biological activity of human IL-17 has been assayed based on its ability to induce the secretion of IL-6 or IL-8 from several lines of human fibroblasts.[112,113] Murine IL-17 can be similarly assayed by its ability to induce the secretion of IL-6 from NIH/3T3 murine fibroblasts.

1. Induction of IL-6 secretion by human fibroblasts

Materials and reagents

- Human fibroblast cell line (e.g., human foreskin fibroblasts [ATCC Cat. No. CRL-1635] or MRC-5 human lung fibroblasts [ATCC Cat. No. CCL-171])
- Recombinant human IL-17 standard
- Culture medium as indicated for the cell line used (e.g., Eagle's MEM containing 10% heat-inactivated FCS, 1.5 g/l sodium bicarbonate,

and supplemented with 2 m*M* L-glutamine, 100 U/ml penicillin, 100 μg/ml streptomycin, 0.1 m*M* nonessential amino acids, and 1 m*M* sodium pyruvate)

- Washing buffer: PBS containing 1% FCS (filter-sterilized)
- 96-well tissue culture plates (flat bottom)
- Pasteur pipettes
- Refrigerated centrifuge (set at 4°C)
- CO_2 incubator (humidified, set at 37°C and 5% CO_2)
- ELISA kit for IL-6

Protocol

(*Note*: All materials and reagents must be sterile and proper aseptic techniques must be used when handling the cells.)

1. Harvest the fibroblast by trypsinization, and wash twice with cold washing buffer and once with complete medium. Count and resuspend the cells in culture medium to 1×10^5 cells/ml. Add 200 μl of the cell suspension per well in a 96-well plate.
2. Dilute samples and standards (0.1 to 10 ng/ml) in culture medium. Add 50 μl of each dilution per well. Assay in triplicate. Include a negative control containing medium alone.
3. Incubate for 48 hr at 37°C in a 5% CO_2 atmosphere.
4. Collect the supernatants and store at –80°C until assay.
5. Measure the concentration of IL-6 in the supernantants using an appropriate ELISA.
6. Calculate the IL-17 concentration by comparison to rIL-17 standard curve. Calculate the sample concentration by comparison to standard curve and multiplication by dilution factor.

Comments

1. Samples containing mixtures of cytokines should be retested in the presence of blocking anti-IL-17 antibodies.
2. The presence of TNFα or IFNγ potentiates the effect of IL-17.
3. Murine IL-17 can be assayed by measuring its ability to induce IL-6 production on NIH/3T3 fibroblasts.

P. Interleukin-18

Interleukin-18 (IL-18) is a cytokine that shares some common biological activities with IL-12 and structural similarities with the IL-1 family of proteins.[114,115] In fact, it was originally known as Interferon-γ-inducing factor (IGIF) or IL-1γ. IL-18 is produced by a variety of cells, including Kupfer cells, monocytes, keratinocytes, osteoblasts, and adrenal cortex. Although IL-18 is a pleiotropic cytokine, its more recognized activity is the induction of secretion of IFNγ by peripheral blood mononuclear cells.[114,115] In addition, IL-18 has costimulatory activities on Th1 cells, including the enhancement of Th1 cytokine production and Fas-ligand expression, and it induces IFNγ secretion by activated B cells with a concomitant decrease in IgE production.[116,117] The ability of IL-18 to induce IFNγ secretion on mononuclear cells has been used as the basis of a bioassay. Normally, a human myelomonocytic cell line (KG-1) or ConA-activated murine lymphocytes are incubated with IL-18-containing samples and the supernatants are later assayed for their content of IFNγ by ELISA.

1. *IFNγ induction assay for human IL-18*

Materials and reagents

- Human myelomonocytic leukemia cells, KG-1 (ATCC Cat. No. CRL-8031)
- Recombinant (human) IL-18 standard
- Culture medium: RPMI-1640 containing 10% heat-inactivated FCS and supplemented with 2 m*M* L-glutamine, 10 m*M* HEPES, 100 U/ml penicillin, 100 μg/ml streptomycin, 50 μM 2-mercaptoethanol, and 1 m*M* sodium pyruvate
- Washing buffer: PBS containing 1% FCS (filter-sterilized)
- 96-well tissue culture plates (flat bottom)
- 15- and 50-ml centrifuge tubes
- Pasteur pipettes
- Refrigerated centrifuge (set at 4°C)
- CO_2 incubator (humidified, set at 37°C and 5% CO_2)
- ELISA kit for IFNγ

Protocol

(*Note*: All materials and reagents must be sterile and proper aseptic techniques must be used when handling the cells.)

1. Culture KG-1 cells in at a density of 3×10^5 cells/ml in culture medium for 4 days.
2. Adjust cell density to 3×10^6 cells/ml. Using a 96-well plate, add 100 μl/well.
3. Dilute samples and standards (0.01 to 10 ng/ml) with culture medium. Test each dilution in triplicate, including a negative control containing medium only. Add 100 μl per well.
4. Incubate at 37°C and 5% CO_2 for 24 hr.
5. Remove the supernatant and store at –70°C until assay.
6. Assay supernatants for human IFNγ by ELISA.
7. Calculate the IL-18 concentration. Plot standard IL-18 concentration on the *x*-axis vs. IFNγ production on the *y*-axis. Calculate the sample concentration by comparison to standard curve and multiplication by dilution factor.

Comments

1. Specificity for IL-18 needs to be demonstrated by inhibition with blocking anti-IL-18 monoclonal antibodies.
2. Murine IL-18 can be similarly assayed using cultures of ConA-activated T lymphocytes.

Q. *Tumor necrosis factors*

Tumor necrosis factor-α (TNFα) and tumor necrosis factor-β (TNFβ, lymphotoxin) are two pleiotropic cytokines secreted primarily by monocyte/macrophages and T lymphocytes, respectively.[118] TNFα was originally described as a factor present in the serum of *Bacillus Calmette-Guerin* (BCG)-treated mice that induced tumor necrosis in tumor-bearing mice.[119] Although there is only a moderate degree of homology between TNFα and TNFβ, both forms bind to the same receptors and elicit similar activities.[118,120] TNFα is the principal mediator of natural immunity against Gram-negative bacteria and a key mediator of inflammatory responses and septic shock.[118] In addition, TNFα/β have many other activities, including a cytotoxic effect toward certain target cells and tumors, induction of MHC class I and II molecules on target cells, activation of polymorphonuclear leukocytes, induction of expression of adherence molecules on endothelial cells, and co-stimulatory effects of T and B lymphocytes.[2,118,120] Extracellular forms of TNF receptors are shed and appear in biological fluids, potentially acting as regulators of TNF activity.[121-123]

Bioassays for TNFα/β are based on its cytotoxic effect toward target cells such as murine L929 fibroblasts[124] and WEHI-164 fibrosarcoma cell line.[125] Although these bioassays detect both human and mouse TNF activity, they do not differentiate between TNFα and TNFβ.

1. *L929 cytotoxicity assay for TNFα/β*

Materials and reagents

- Murine L929 fibroblasts (TNF-sensitive)
- Recombinant TNFα or TNFβ standards (human or mouse)
- Actinomycin D (Sigma Cat. No. A-9415)
- Culture medium: RPMI-1640 containing 10% heat-inactivated FCS and supplemented with 2 m*M* L-glutamine, 10 m*M* HEPES, 100 U/ml penicillin, 100 μg/ml streptomycin, 50 μ*M* 2-mercaptoethanol, and 1 m*M* sodium pyruvate
- Porcine trypsin solution (Sigma Cat. No. T-4549)
- Washing buffer: PBS containing 1% FCS (filter-sterilized)
- Reagents necessary for MTT proliferation assay (see Chapter 3)
- 8-well aspirator (e.g., Drummond, CMS)
- 96-well tissue culture plates (flat bottom)

- 15- and 50-ml centrifuge tubes
- Pasteur pipettes
- Refrigerated centrifuge (set at 4°C)
- CO_2 incubator (humidified, set at 37°C and 5% CO_2)
- Multi-well spectrophotometer (ELISA reader)

Protocol

(Note: All materials and reagents must be sterile and proper aseptic techniques must be used when handling the cells.)

1. On day 1, harvest L929 fibroblasts by trypsinization (see protocol below). Remove trypsin by washing cells once in 20 ml cold culture medium. Centrifuge the cells at 200*g* for 10 min, count, and resuspend in culture medium to a cell density of 4×10^5 cells/ml.
2. Using a 96-well tissue culture plate, add 100 µl of the fibroblast suspension per well and incubate overnight at 37°C and 5% CO_2. Set one horizontal row for each sample to be tested, plus one for the standards.
3. Next day, check the cells with an inverted microscope. Under these conditions, cells should be confluent. Using an 8-channel aspirator, aspirate the medium from the wells.
4. Dilute samples and standards (serial twofold dilutions) in culture medium. Add 50 µl of each dilution per well, starting with column 2. Add 50 µl of medium alone to column 1 (medium control).
5. Add 50 µl/well of a 2-µg/ml solution of actinomycin D in culture medium. Incubate the plates for 18 hr at 37°C and 5% CO_2.
6. Add 10 µl per well of a 5 mg/ml solution of MTT in PBS. Return to the incubator and incubate for 4 additional hours.
7. Remove supernatants from the wells with an 8-channel aspirator. Add 100 µl per well of acidic isopropanol (0.04 *N* HCl in isopropanol). Mix well until all crystals are dissolved.
8. Read on a multi-well spectrophotometer using a test wavelength of 570 nm and a reference wavelength of 630 nm. Read plates within 1 hr of addition of the acidic isopropanol. (Refer to Chapter 3 for MTT assay.)
9. Using semilog paper, plot OD_{570} (on *y*-axis) vs. the standard concentration (on the *x*-axis). Calculate the TNF concentration in unknown samples by referring to standard curve and multiplying by the dilution factor. Alternatively, calculation can also be performed by calculating the dilution of sample giving 50% of maximal lysis and comparing that to the standard dilution at which 50% maximal lysis occurs.

Comments

1. L929 cells from different sources may vary widely in their sensitivity to TNF. It is better to obtain cells whose TNF sensitivity is known.

2. Several modifications to the original MTT proliferation assay are discussed in Chapter 3. The extraction reagent (acidic isopropanol) can be substituted for 10% SDS (pH 4.5) or other reagents to minimize protein precipitation if it interferes with spectrophotometric readings.

2. Maintenance and passage of L929 cells

Materials and reagents

- L929 fibroblasts
- Diluted porcine trypsin solution (Sigma Cat. No. T-4549)
- Culture medium: RPMI-1640 containing 10% heat-inactivated FCS and supplemented with 2 m*M* L-glutamine, 10 m*M* HEPES, 100 U/ml penicillin, 100 μg/ml streptomycin, 50 μ*M* 2-mercaptoethanol, and 1 m*M* sodium pyruvate
- 75-cm^2 tissue culture flasks
- 15- and 50-ml centrifuge tubes
- Pasteur pipettes
- Refrigerated centrifuge (set at 4°C)
- CO_2 incubator (humidified, set at 37°C and 5% CO_2)

Protocol

(*Note*: All materials and reagents must be sterile and proper aseptic techniques must be used when handling the cells.)

1. Seed fibroblasts at an initial density of 4 × 10^5 cells/ml in culture medium.
2. Incubate at 37°C and 5% CO_2 until the cells reach confluence (~5 to 7 days). The medium can be discarded and replaced on day 4.
3. For subculture, aspirate the medium and add 3 ml (for a 75-cm^2 flask) of a trypsin solution. Incubate at 37°C for approximately 1 to 2 min or until cells start to detach from the flask.
4. Shake the flask and transfer the cells with a sterile pipettete into a 50-ml centrifuge tube containing 20 ml culture medium at 4°C. Resuspend in culture medium and count. The cells are ready for subculture or assay.

R. Interferons

Interferons (IFN) are a group of cytokines with the ability to inhibit viral replication *in vitro*.[2] Interferons have been divided into two main groups: Type I or viral interferon, including IFNα (leukocyte derived) and IFNβ (fibroblast derived); and Type II or immune interferon, including IFNγ, which is produced mainly by T lymphocytes as a result of antigenic or mitogenic stimulation.[126] IFNα and IFNβ have similar activities and bind to the same membrane receptors,[127] whereas IFNγ, which displays a different set of immunoregulatory activities, binds to a different receptor.[128] The activities of IFNγ are many and include induction of expression of MHC class I and II molecules on a variety of target cells, macrophage activation, increased cytotoxicity in NK cells and CTLs, inhibition of many IL-4-mediated functions, and effects on B cell differentiation.[129]

Interferons, in general, can be assayed based on their antiviral activity.[130] This assay, however, does not distinguish among the different types of IFN, although with the use of specific neutralizing antibodies, this may be possible. In addition, several bioassays not based on antiviral activity have been reported for the detection and quantification of IFNγ. Some of these assays include the induction of class II MHC molecule expression on target cells,[131] induction of microbicidal activity,[132] and cytotoxicity against target cells such as the murine B lymphoma cell line WEHI-279.[133]

1. Antiviral activity assay for interferons α, β, and γ

The basis for this assay is the antiviral effect induced by all interferons. In this assay, murine L929 fibroblasts are cultured in the presence of vesicular stomatitis virus (VSV) and dilutions of IFN-containing samples and standards. Measurement of IFN activity is then based on the inhibition of the cytopathic effect (cell lysis). This assay employs the MTT reduction assay to quantitate the extent of cell death.

Materials and reagents

- Murine L929 fibroblasts (IFN-sensitive)
- Vesicular stomatitis virus (VSV, Indiana strain; ATCC)
- Recombinant IFNα, β, or γ standard (mouse)
- Culture medium: Eagle minimum essential medium (EMEM), containing 5% FCS, 15 m*M* HEPES, 100 U/ml penicillin, 100 μg/ml streptomycin
- Trypsin solution (Sigma Cat. No. T-4549)
- Reagents needed for MTT assay (see Chapter 3)
- 8-well aspirator (e.g., Drummond, CMS)
- 96-well tissue culture plates
- 75-cm² tissue culture flasks
- 15- and 50-ml centrifuge tubes
- Pasteur pipettes
- Refrigerated centrifuge (set at 4°C)
- CO_2 incubator (humidified, set at 37°C and 5% CO_2)

Protocol

(*Note*: All materials and reagents must be sterile and proper aseptic techniques must be used when handling the cells.)

1. Harvest L929 cells after they have reached confluence (see protocol for maintenance of L929 cells, Section Q in this chapter). Seed enough cells into a new flask so that they will again be confluent in 24 hr (~1:2 dilution in culture medium). Use these "new" cells for the assay.
2. Harvest the cells by trypsinization. Wash 3× in culture medium to remove the trypsin. Centrifuge at 200*g* for 10 min, count, and resuspend to a cell density of 1.5×10^5 cells/ml in culture medium.
3. Add 100 μl of medium to each well. Allow one row for each sample and one for the standards.
4. Add 50 μl of sample to the third well in each row. Prepare serial threefold dilutions by mixing and transferring 50 μl to the next well (well # 4) and repeating until well # 12. Discard the last 50 μl. The first two wells are reserved for controls: cells alone (well # 1) and cells plus virus without sample (well # 2).
5. Add 100 μl of the fibroblast suspension to each well, except for a well reserved as a blank.
6. Incubate the cells for 24 hr at 37°C and 5% CO_2.
7. On the next day, dilute the VSV suspension in culture medium to 10^3 PFU/ml.
8. Aspirate medium from the wells using an 8-channel aspirator. Add 200 μl of the virus suspension to all wells except for the first column (cells only). Add 200 μl culture medium to these wells instead.
9. Incubate the plates at 37°C and 5% CO_2 for at least 24 hr. Observe the cells under an inverted microscope to determine the amount of cell destruction. Cells cultured with VSV in the absence of IFN should be 75 to 90% destroyed.
10. Using an 8-channel aspirator, aspirate the supernatant from the plates into a flask containing bleach. Add 80 μl per well of culture medium and 20 μl per well of a 5-mg/ml MTT solution in PBS, except for the blank.
11. Incubate for 4 hr at 37°C and 5% CO_2, and then add 100 μl per well of an acidic isopropanol solution. Mix and allow crystals to dissolve. (Refer to Chapter 3 for MTT proliferation assay.)
12. Read on a multiwell scanning spectrophotometer using a test wavelength of 570 nm and a reference wavelength of 630 nm. Read plates within 1 hr of addition of the acidic isopropanol. Use the blank for zeroing the spectrophotometer.
13. Calculate the IFN concentration. Plot OD_{570} (*y*-axis) as a function of standard IFN concentration (*x*-axis). Calculate the IFN concentration in unknown samples by referring to the standard curve and multiplying by the dilution factor. Alternatively, calculation can also be performed by calculating the dilution of sample giving 50% of maximal lysis and comparing that to the standard dilution at which 50% maximal lysis occurs.

Comments

1. As with TNFα, the sensitivity of L929 cells from different sources to IFN varies widely. Obtain cells of known sensitivity.
2. The appropriate dose of virus is crucial to the sensitivity and reproducibility of the assay. An appropriate dose should give detachment of 75 to 90% of cells after 24 hr. It is advisable to titrate virus pools to determine the optimal challenge dose.
3. VSV is a potentially pathogenic virus. Appropriate care and technique should be used when handling the virus or VSV-containing cultures.
4. As interferons are species specific, this assay detects murine but not human IFN. The bioassay for human IFN can be performed almost identically with the exception of using susceptible human cell lines and recombinant human IFN standards. Some human cell lines used with VSV include WISH, a human amnion epithelial cell line (ATCC Cat. No. CCL 25); and AG-1732 and GM-2504A, a pair of human skin fibroblast cell lines.[134]
5. Stocks of VSV are generated from the supernatants of infected L929 or Vero cells. Supernatants are aliquoted and stored frozen at –70°C. The potency of the virus stock is determined by a plaque assay method.[126]

2. WEHI-279 cell cytotoxicity assay for murine IFNγ

This assay is based on the ability of IFNγ to inhibit the proliferation of the murine B lymphoma cell line WEHI-279.[133] The indicator cells are cultured in the presence of IFNγ-containing samples or standards, and the inhibition of proliferation is assessed by [^{3}H-methyl] thymidine incorporation.

Materials and reagents

- WEHI-279 cells (ATCC Cat. No. CRL-1704)
- Recombinant murine IFNγ standard
- Culture medium: RPMI-1640 containing 10% heat-inactivated FCS and supplemented with 2 m*M* L-glutamine, 10 m*M* HEPES, 100 U/ml penicillin, 100 μg/ml streptomycin, 50 μ*M* 2-mercaptoethanol, and 1 m*M* sodium pyruvate
- Washing buffer: PBS containing 1% FCS (filter-sterilized)
- [^{3}H-methyl] thymidine
- 96-well tissue culture plates (flat bottom)
- 15- and 50-ml centrifuge tubes
- Pasteur pipettes
- Refrigerated centrifuge (set at 4°C)

- CO_2 incubator (humidified, set at 37°C and 5% CO_2)
- Cell harvester (e.g., Skatron)
- Glass fiber filter mats (Skatron)
- Scintillation vials
- Scintillation cocktail (e.g., Econo-Safe, Research Products International)
- Scintillation counter

Protocol

(*Note*: All materials and reagents must be sterile and proper aseptic techniques must be used when handling the cells.)

1. Harvest the WEHI-279 cells. Wash twice with 20 ml cold washing buffer, centrifuging at 200*g* for 10 min. Count the cells and resuspend in culture medium to a density of 4×10^5 cells/ml.
2. Dilute samples and standards (0.1 to 100 U/ml) in culture medium. Add 50 μl/well. Include a control containing medium alone. Assay each dilution in triplicate.
3. Add 50 μl/well of the indicator cell suspension. Incubate for 24 hr at 37°C and 5% CO_2.
4. Add 20 μl/well of a 50-μCi/ml solution of [^{3}H-methyl] thymidine in culture medium (final concentration is 1 μCi/well) during the last 4 to 6 hr of incubation.
5. Harvest the cells onto glass fiber mats with the aid of a cell harvester. Determine [^{3}H-methyl] thymidine uptake by liquid scintillation counting.
6. Calculate the IFNγ concentration by comparison to IFNγ standard curve. Using semilog or probit paper, plot standard IFNγ concentration on the *x*-axis vs. proliferation (in cpm) on the *y*-axis. Calculate the sample concentration by comparison to standard curve and multiplication by dilution factor.

Comments

1. WEHI-279 cells are maintained by culture in RPMI-10% FCS medium. Seed flask at an initial density of 5×10^4 cells/ml. Subculture every third day or when the cells reach an approximate density of 1×10^6 cells/ml. Culturing cells at higher densities will result in decreased cell viability and potential changes in their sensitivity to IFNγ.
2. The sensitivity of WEHI-279 cells to IFNγ may decrease after prolonged culture. It is advisable to keep aliquots of frozen cells so fresh cultures can be started if such is the case.
3. As with other cytokines, results should be confirmed by demonstrating inhibition in the presence of neutralizing anti-IFNγ antibodies.

3. *Induction of expression of MHC class II antigens*

In this bioassay, IFNγ is quantitated based on its ability to induce expression of MHC class II antigens on appropriate target cells (the myelomonocytic cell line WEHI-3 for murine IFNγ assays, and the colon adenocarcinoma cell line COLO-205 for human IFNγ assays).[135] Cells are cultured in the presence of IFNγ-containing samples or standards and the expression of MHC class II molecules is then evaluated by flow cytometry.

Materials and reagents

- COLO-205 (ATCC Cat. No. CCL 1222) or WEHI-3 cells (ATCC Cat. No. TIB 68)
- Recombinant human or murine IFNγ standards
- Culture medium: RPMI-1640 containing 10% heat-inactivated FCS and supplemented with 2 m*M* L-glutamine, 10 m*M* HEPES, 100 U/ml penicillin, 100 μg/ml streptomycin, 50 μ*M* 2-mercaptoethanol, and 1 m*M* sodium pyruvate
- Washing buffer: PBS containing 1% FCS (filter-sterilized)
- Biotinylated antibodies specific for human HLA-DR (nonpolymorphic determinant) or murine I-A^d (e.g., BD Pharmingen)
- Avidin or streptavidin-fluorescein isothiocyanate (Av-FITC)
- PBS-1% FCS containing 10 m*M* NaN_3
- PBS-1% heat-inactivated normal mouse serum containing 10 m*M* NaN_3
- 24-well tissue culture plates
- 12 × 75-mm centrifuge tubes
- 15- and 50-ml centrifuge tubes
- Pasteur pipettes
- Sterile rubber policeman
- Refrigerated centrifuge (set at 4°C)
- CO_2 incubator (humidified, set at 37°C and 5% CO_2)
- Tabletop centrifuge
- Reagents and equipment for flow cytometry (see Chapter 2)

Protocol

(*Note*: All materials and reagents must be sterile and proper aseptic techniques must be used when handling the cells. The protocol for cell staining does not require sterility.)

1. Harvest indicator cells and resuspend them in culture medium to a density of 5 × 10^5 cells/ml.
2. Dilute samples and standards (1 to 100 U/ml) in culture medium. Test four to five different dilutions. Add 0.5 ml of the diluted samples/standards to each well of a 24-well tissue culture plate. Add 0.5

ml medium alone to two control wells (one for background staining and one for basal MHC class II expression).

3. Add 0.5 ml medium and 1.0 ml of the indicator cell suspension per well. Incubate for 48 hr at 37°C and 5% CO_2.
4. Harvest the cells in each well by gently scraping with a rubber policeman and pipetting the cell suspension up and down several times with a Pasteur pipette. Transfer the cells to a 12 × 75-mm centrifuge tube and pellet the cells by centrifugation at 200*g* for 10 min at 4°C.
5. Aspirate the supernatants by suction and wash the cells twice with ice-cold PBS-1% FCS containing 10 m*M* NaN_3. After the last wash, resuspend the cells in 100 µl of PBS containing heat-inactivated normal mouse serum and 10 m*M* NaN_3. Incubate for 30 minutes on ice.
6. Add 20 µl of biotinylated anti-MHC class II antibody to each tube, except for the background staining control. Antibodies should be diluted in PBS-1% FCS containing 10 m*M* NaN_3 according to the manufacturer's recommendations or optimal staining concentrations should be determined beforehand. Normally, a final antibody concentration of 5 to 10 µg/ml gives adequate results.
7. Incubate the tubes for 60 min on ice. Wash twice with ice-cold PBS-1% FCS containing 10 m*M* NaN_3 and resuspend in 100 µl of the same buffer. Add avidin-FITC conjugate diluted according to manufacturer's recommendations.
8. Incubate for 30 min on ice. Wash twice with cold PBS-1% FCS containing 10 m*M* NaN_3 and resuspend in 0.5 ml of the same buffer. Maintain samples on ice until analysis.
9. Quantitate cellular fluorescence by flow cytometry as described in Chapter 2.
10. Construct a standard curve by plotting mean fluorescence intensity (MFI) as a function of the IFNγ concentration. Calculate the IFNγ concentration in samples by reference to standard curve.

Comments

1. Other indicator cell lines can also be used. IFNγ is species specific; thus, the samples and the standards need to be assayed on indicator cells of the same species.
2. Antibodies directed against MHC class II (mouse or human) can be obtained from a variety of commercial sources. Alternatively, several hybridomas secreting anti-MHC class II antibodies are available from the ATCC.
3. If samples cannot be analyzed on the same day, they can be fixed with 1% paraformaldehyde and kept at 4°C.

Table 6.1 summarizes the different indicator cell lines used for the cytokine bioassays, the species specificity of the assay, and potentially interfering

Table 6.1 Indicator Cell Lines Used in Cytokine Bioassays: Species Specificity and Interfering Cytokines

Assay	Indicator Cell	Species Specificity		Interfering Cytokines
		Human	Mouse	
IL-1α/β	Thymocytes (C3H/HeJ)	Yes	Yes	IL-2, IL-6, TNFα
	D10.G4.1	Yes	Yes	IL-2, IL-4
IL-2	HT-2, CTLL-2	Yes	Yes	IL-4, IL-15
IL-3	MC/9	No	Yes	IL-4, SCF
	TF-1	Yes	No	IL-4, IL-5, IL-6, IL-13, GM-CSF, EPO
IL-4	HT-2, CTLL-2	No	Yes	IL-2, IL-15
	CT.4S	No	Yes	IL-2 (high conc.)
	CTLL-hu IL-4R	Yes	Yes	IL-2, IL-15
IL-5	Splenocytes + dextran-SO_4	?	Yes	?
	BCL_1	Yes	Yes	IL-2
	TF-1	Yes	No	IL-3, IL-4, IL-6, IL-13, GM-CSF, EPO
IL-6	B9, 7TD1	Yes	Yes	IL-4 (high conc.)
IL-7	2E8	Yes	Yes	?
IL-8	Human neutrophils	Yes	No	Other chemokines
IL-9	M-07e	Yes	Yes	IL-3, GM-CSF
IL-10	Th1 clones (murine)	Yes	Yes	IL-4, TGFβ, IFNγ
	MC/9	Yes	Yes	IL-3, IL-4, SCF
IL-11	T1165, T10	Yes	Yes	IL-6
IL-12	PBMC (human)	Yes	Yes	IL-2, IL-4, IL-7, IL-18, IFNγ
IL-13	B9	Yes	Yes	IL-6, IL-4 (high conc.)
IL-15	CTLL-2	Yes	Yes	IL-2, IL-4
IL-16	$CD4^+$ T cells	Yes	Yes	Several chemokines
	HUT 78	Yes	No	IL-2, IL-15
IL-17	HFF, MRC-5	Yes	No	IL-6, TNFα, IFNγ
	NIH/3T3	Yes	Yes	IL-6, TNFα, IFNγ
IL-18	KG-1	Yes	?	IL-12, IFNγ
	ConA blasts	Yes	Yes	IL-12, IFNγ
TNFα/β	L929	Yes	Yes	?
IFNs	L929 + VSV	No	Yes	TNFα/β
(α/β/γ)	WISH + VSV	Yes	No	?
IFNγ	WEHI-279	No	Yes	?
	WEHI-3	No	Yes	?
	COLO-205	Yes	No	?

cytokines. This table indicates the cytokine bioassay, the indicator cell lines, whether the indicator cell line can be used to assay the human and/or murine cytokine, and cytokines that may potentially interfere with the bioassay, either through stimulation or inhibition. Note that species specificity needs to be taken into consideration with interfering cytokines (i.e., murine IL-4 interferes with the IL-2 bioassay using murine CTLL-2 cells; however, human IL-4 does not interfere because human IL-4 is not active on murine cells).

III. Immunoassays

Under this description are assays that are based on the detection and quantification of cytokines based on their reactivity with specific antibodies (monoclonal and/or polyclonal) or binding to specific cytokine receptors. These assays have become the preferred method for cytokine quantitation, primarily because of their speed and specificity. Unlike the bioassays, which depend on the measurement of the biological response of indicator cells, immunoassays are based on immunogenicity and thus are inherently very specific, especially when monoclonal antibodies are used. The main advantages and disadvantages of immunoassays are listed below.

Advantages

1. Very specific (differentiate between cytokine subtypes) and reproducible
2. Fast (results are normally obtained in 3 to 4 hr)
3. Not susceptible to potentiation or inhibition by other cytokines
4. Generally less susceptible than bioassays to interference by cytokine antagonists or soluble cytokine receptors (depends on the antibodies used for capture and detection)

Disadvantages

1. May not differentiate between biologically active and inactive cytokines
2. Sometimes less sensitive than bioassays (~50 pg/ml)
3. Relatively expensive (especially if relying on commercially available kits)

Although several formats have been employed in the immunoassay of cytokines, perhaps the most common is the "sandwich-type" ELISA, in which two different anti-cytokine antibodies (monoclonal and/or polyclonal) are used for capture and detection, respectively. Quantification is then based on the spectrophotometric determination of enzymatic activity linked to the detecting antibody. Because the technique is basically the same for any cytokine, with exception of the antibodies, only a "generic" method is described here. However, as properties (e.g., affinity, avidity) of different antibodies may vary, the conditions for a particular assay may have to be optimized for best results.

Monoclonal and polyclonal anti-cytokine antibodies can be purchased in purified form from a variety of companies (see Tables 6.2 and 6.3), or the hybridomas can be obtained from the ATCC, grown in the laboratory and the antibodies purified (see Chapter 9). For cytokine immunoassays, two different monoclonal antibodies or a monoclonal and a polyclonal antibody can be combined for use in an ELISA. Alternatively, appropriate monoclonal or polyclonal antibodies can also be used for neutralization purposes in bioassays. Companies such as BD Pharmingen, R & D Systems, and Biosource International offer blocking antibodies suitable for cytokine-neutralization studies in tissue culture, and pairs of monoclonal antibodies suitable for use in ELISAs, with the advantage that the detection antibody is sold already biotinylated.

Table 6.2 Monoclonal Anti-Mouse Cytokine Antibodies

Assay	Capture	Detection	Blocking
IL-2	JES6-1A12	JES6-5H4	S4B6
IL-3	MP2-8F8	MP2-43D11	MP2-8F8
IL-4	11B11, BVD4-1D11	BVD6-24G2, BVD4-1D11	11B11
IL-5	TRFK-5	TRFK-4	TRFK-5
IL-6	MP5-20F3	MP5-32C11	MP5-20F3
IL-9	D8402E8	D9302C12	D9302C12
IL-10	JES5-2A5	SXC-1	JES5-2A5, SCX-1
IL-12	9A5 (p70)	C17.8 (p40)	C17.8
IL-17	TC11-18H10.1	TC11-8H4.1	
GM-CSF	MP1-22E9	MP1-31G6	MP1-22E9
TNFα	MP6-XT22	MP6-XT3	MP6-XT3
IFNγ	R4-6A2	XMG1.2	R4-6A2, XMG1.2

Note: Many of these antibodies can be obtained from commercial sources, such as BD Pharmingen, R & D Systems, or BioSource International, to name a few. Some hybridomas are also available through the ATCC. Additional monoclonal and polyclonal anti-cytokine antibodies are also available from other vendors. This table is intended for reference purposes only and does not imply endorsement of any specific company by the authors.

A. *General protocol for cytokine ELISA*

Materials and reagents

- Enhanced protein-binding plates (e.g., Immulon-2, Dynatech, Chantilly, VA)
- Multichannel pipette (50 to 200 μl)
- Parafilm™
- Refrigerator
- Incubator (37°C)
- Multiwell spectrophotometer (ELISA Reader)
- Capture and detection anti-cytokine antibodies (detection antibody is biotinylated)

Table 6.3 Monoclonal Anti-Human Cytokine Antibodies

Assay	Capture	Detection	Blocking
IL-1α	36-3B3-14	28.9	28.9
IL-1β	ILB1-H6	ILB1-H21 ILB1-H67	
IL-2	5344.111	B33-2	MQ1-17H12
IL-3	BVD8-3G11	BVD3-1F9	BVD8-3G11
IL-4	8D4-8	MP4-25D2	MP4-25D2
IL-5	TRFK-5	JES1-5A10	JES1-5A10
IL-6	MQ2-13A5	MQ2-39C3	MQ2-13A5
IL-7	BVD10-40F6	BVD10-11C10	BVD10-40F6
IL-10	JES3-9D7	JES3-12G8	JES3-9D7
IL-12	C8.3 (p40/p70)	C8.6	C8.6
IL-13	JES10-35G12	JES10-2E10	JES10-5E2
IL-15	G243-935	G243-886	
GM-CSF	BVD2-23B6	BVD2-21C11	BVD2-23B6
TNFα	MAb1	MAb11	MAb1
IFNγ	NIB42	4S.B3	NIB42

Note: Many of these antibodies can be obtained from commercial sources, such BD Pharmingen, R & D Systems or BioSource International, to name a few. Some hybridomas are also available through the ATCC. Additional monoclonal and polyclonal anti-cytokine antibodies are also available from other vendors. This table is intended for reference purposes only and does not imply endorsement of any specific company by the authors.

- Avidin (or streptavidin)-alkaline phosphatase (or peroxidase) conjugate (e.g., Jackson Immunoresearch, Sigma, etc.)
- Substrate:
  - p-Nitrophenylphosphate tablets (Sigma Cat. No. N-2640) for alkaline phosphatase
  - 2,2′-Azino-*bis*(3-ethylbenzthiazoline-6-sulfonic acid) (ATBS, Sigma Cat. No. A-1888) for horseradish peroxidase
- Coating buffer: 0.1 *M* $NaHCO_3$, pH 8.2
- Blocking buffer: Phosphate-buffered saline containing 10% FCS (PBS-10% FCS) or PBS containing 1% bovine serum albumin and 2% normal rat serum
- Dilution buffer: PBS-10% FCS or PBS containing 1% bovine serum albumin and 5% normal rat serum
- Washing buffer: PBS containing 0.05% Tween 20 (PBS-Tween)
- Substrate solution:
  - For alkaline phosphatase, dissolve *p*-nitrophenyl phosphate tablets to a final concentration of 1 mg/ml in 20 m*M* diethanolamine-HCl buffer, pH 9.5, containing 1 m*M* $MgCl_2$
  - For horseradish peroxidase, dissolve ATBS to a final concentration of 0.3 mg/ml in 0.1 *M* citric acid, pH 4.35; then add 10 μl of 30% H_2O_2 per 10 ml of solution.

- Stopping solution:
  - 10 N NaOH for alkaline phosphatase
  - 16% SDS solution in 40% N,N-dimethylformamide (SDS/DMF) for peroxidase

1. Coating plates with capture antibody

1. Dilute purified anti-cytokine antibody to 1 to 2 μg/ml in coating buffer.
2. Using enhanced protein-binding plates (e.g., Immulon-2, Dynatech), add 100 μl of the diluted antibody per well.
3. Seal the plate with Parafilm™ and incubate for 6 hr at room temperature or overnight at 4°C.

2. Blocking the plates

1. Discard the antibody solution and wash the wells twice with PBS.
2. Add 200 μl/well of blocking buffer.
3. Seal the plate with Parafilm and incubate for a minimum of 2 hr at 37°C or overnight at 4°C.
4. Plates can be used immediately after completion of the blocking step, or stored at 4°C without removing the blocking solution. If stored for later use, it is recommended to place the sealed plates inside plastic bags (e.g., Ziplock™ bags) to minimize evaporation.

3. Samples/standards

1. Determine the number of wells needed. It is advisable to assay each sample at least in duplicate or triplicate. Include extra wells for blanks and recombinant cytokine standards (six or seven different concentrations in the 10 to 2000 pg/ml range). (See Comment 3.)
2. Add samples and standards (50 μl/well). Cover and incubate for at least 2 hr at 37°C or overnight at 4°C. (See Comment 4.)
3. Wash 4× with PBS-0.05% Tween 20 (Polyoxyylene-sorbitan monolaureate).

4. Secondary (detection) antibody

1. Dilute the biotinylated secondary (detection) antibody to 1 to 2 μg/ml in dilution buffer. (See comment 5.)
2. Add 60 μl of diluted antibody per well, cover, and incubate for at least 1 hr at 37°C.
3. Wash six times with PBS-0.05% Tween 20.

5. Avidin-enzyme conjugate

1. Dilute the avidin-alkaline phosphatase (or alternatively avidin-peroxidase) conjugate to the manufacturer's recommended dilution (usually 1 to 2 μg/ml) using dilution buffer. (See Comment 6.)
2. Add 100 μl per well, cover, and incubate for at least 30 minutes at 37°C.
3. Wash 6× with PBS-Tween 20.

6. Substrate

1. Prepare the appropriate substrate solution (*p*-nitrophenyl phosphate for alkaline phosphatase, ATBS-H_2O_2 for peroxidase) at least 5 min before use. Substrate solution must be at room temperature.
2. Add 100 μl per well. Allow color to develop at room temperature for 10 to 60 min.
3. Stop the reaction by addition of stop reagent (25 μl/well of 10 *N* NaOH for alkaline-phosphatase reactions, or 100 μl/well of SDS/DMF solution for peroxidase reactions).
4. Read at OD 405 nm.

7. Calculation

1. For manual calculation, construct a standard curve by plotting standard concentration (log scale) in pg/ml against OD_{405}. Calculate sample concentration by comparing sample OD_{405} with the standard curve.
2. A number of computer programs are available for computer-assisted calculation.

Comments

1. In the authors' laboratory, PBS has given satisfactory results as a coating buffer when using enhanced protein-binding plates (e.g., Immulon-2, Dynatech).
2. In the authors' experience, the use of 2 to 5% normal rat serum in both the blocking and diluting buffers has provided good results in minimizing background on cytokine ELISAs based on rat monoclonal antibodies.
3. Standards should be diluted in a buffer that closely matches the composition of the actual samples (e.g., culture media, serum, etc.).
4. The authors have determined that incubation of samples at 37°C rather than 4°C minimizes interference by soluble cytokine receptors, probably due to faster dissociation rates at higher temperatures.

5. The detection antibody may either be purchased already biotinylated or biotinylated in the laboratory (see Chapter 2). Alternatively, the secondary antibody may be used without biotinylation, in which case a biotinylated or enzyme-conjugated third antibody directed against the second antibody (usually anti-immunoglobulin antibody) will be used.
6. Azide is a potent inhibitor of peroxidase; consequently, azide-free buffers should be used throughout if peroxidase conjugates are used for detection.
7. Monoclonal antibody pairs suitable for use in human and murine cytokine ELISAs are available from a variety of commercial sources.
8. "Kits" for human and murine cytokine measurement are available from several vendors, including:

   Amersham Pharmacia Biotech
   BD Pharmingen
   Bio-Source International
   Endogen
   R & D Systems

(This list does not pretend to be all-inclusive.)

B. *Protocol for enhanced ELISA method*

Although the protocol described above for cytokine ELISAs should prove adequate for normal measurements, increased sensitivity may be preferred under some conditions. Increasing the sensitivity of an ELISA may involve addition of a third step or the use of an amplification reaction. A protocol for such an amplification reaction, originally described by Stanley et al.,[136] is presented here. This protocol is based on the amplification of an alkaline-phosphatase enzymatic reaction and results in approximately a 10- to 20-fold increase in sensitivity.
Substrate reaction:

$$\text{NADPH} \xrightarrow{\text{Alkaline phosphatase}} \text{NADH} + \text{Pi}$$

Amplification reaction:

$$(1)\quad \text{NADH} + \text{INT} - \text{violet} \xrightarrow{\text{Diaphorase}} \text{Formazan (red) NAD}^+$$

$$(2)\quad \text{NAD}^+ + \text{Ethanol} \xrightarrow{\text{Alcohol dehydrogenase}} \text{NADH} + \text{Acetaldehyde}$$

Materials and reagents

- TBS: 50 m*M* Tris-HCl, 150 m*M* NaCl, pH 7.5
- β-NADPH (reduced form; Sigma Cat. No. N-1630)
- Alcohol dehydrogenase (Sigma Cat. No. A-3263)
- Diaphorase suspension (Sigma Cat. No. D-3752)
- *p*-Iodonitrotetrazolium (INT-violet; Sigma Cat. No. I-8377)
- Substrate solution: dissolve 2 mg β-NADPH in 12 ml of 50 m*M* diethanolamine-HCl buffer, pH 9.5, containing 1 m*M* $MgCl_2$
- Amplification solution: first dissolve 2 mg lyophilized alcohol dehydrogenase in 11 ml of 50 m*M* phosphate buffer, pH 7.0; then add 60 μl of diaphorase suspension and 1 ml of a 6-mg/ml solution of *p*-iodonitrotetrazolium violet in 36% ethanol. Filter.
- Stopping solution: 0.3 *M* H_2SO_4

Protocol

1. Follow Sections 1 through 5 as described above for the general protocol for cytokine ELISA using an avidin-alkaline phosphatase conjugate.
2. Wash plates 4× with PBS-Tween 20 and 6× with TBS to remove all phosphate.
3. Prepare the substrate solution at least 10 min before use. Substrate solution must be at room temperature.
4. Add 50 μl of substrate solution per well. Incubate for 5 to 10 min at room temperature.
5. Prepare the amplifier solution at least 10 min before use and make sure solution is at room temperature.
6. Without removing the substrate solution from the wells, add 50 μl of the amplifier solution per well. Allow to develop for 5 to 10 min at room temperature.
7. Stop the reaction by addition of 50 μl per well of a 0.3 *M* H_2SO_4 solution.
8. Measure OD at 490 nm.

Comments

1. Amplifier solution should be colorless or slightly yellow. Discard and prepare again if it develops a pink to red color. Unlike the substrate solution, the amplifier solution does not store well at –20°C and is best prepared fresh.
2. An "ELISA Amplification System" kit based on the same reaction is available from GIBCO-BRL (Cat. No. 9589SA).

References

1. Arai, K., Lee, F., Miyajima, A., Miyatake, S., Arai, N., and Yokota, T., Cytokines: coordinators of immune and inflammatory responses, *Annu. Rev. Biochem.*, 59, 783, 1990.
2. Oppenheim, J.J. and Sklatvala, J., Cytokines and their receptors, in *Clinical Applications of Cytokines: Role in Pathogenesis, Diagnosis and Therapy*, Oppenheim, J.J., Rossio, J., and Gearing, A., Eds., Oxford University Press, New York, 1993, 3.
3. Abbas, A.K., Lichtman, A.H., and Pober, J.S., *Cellular and Molecular Immunology*, 2nd. ed., Saunders, Philadelphia, 1994, 240.
4. Mosmann, T.R., Cherwinski, H., Bond, M.W., Giedlin, M.A., and Coffman, R.L., Two types of murine helper T cell clone. I. Definition according to profiles of lymphokine activities and secreted proteins, *J. Immunol.*, 136, 2348, 1986.
5. Mosmann, T.R. and Coffman, R.L., Th1 and Th2 cells: different patterns of lymphokine secretion lead to different functional properties, *Annu. Rev. Immunol.*, 7, 145, 1989.
6. Rossio, J.L., and Gearing, A.J.H., Measurement of cytokines, in *Clinical Applications of Cytokines: Role in Pathogenesis, Diagnosis and Therapy*, Oppenheim, J.J., Rossio, J., and Gearing, A., Eds., Oxford University Press, New York, 1993, 16.
7. Fernandez-Botran, R. and Vetvicka, V., *Advanced Methods in Cellular Immunology*, CRC Press, Boca Raton, FL, 2000.
8. Watson, J., Continuous proliferation of murine antigen-specific helper T lymphocytes in culture, *J. Exp. Med.*, 150, 1510, 1979.
9. Gillis, S., Ferm, M.M., Ou, W., and Smith, K.A., T cell growth factor: parameters of production and a quantitative microassay for activity, *J. Immunol.*, 120, 2027, 1978.
10. Fernandez-Botran, R., Krammer, P.H., Diamantstein, T., Uhr, J.W., and Vitetta, E.S., B cell-stimulatory factor 1 (BSF-1) promotes growth of helper T cell lines, *J. Exp. Med.*, 164, 580, 1986.
11. Grabstein, K.H., Eisenman, J., Shanebeck, K., Rauch, C., Srinivasan, S., Fung, V., Beers, C., Richardson, J., Schoenborn, M.A., Ahdieh, M., Johnson, L., Alderson, M.R., Watson, J.D., Anderson, D.M., and Giri, J.G., Cloning of a T cell growth factor that interacts with the β chain of the interleukin-2 receptor, *Science*, 264, 965, 1994.
12. Dinarello, C.A., Biology of interleukin-1, *FASEB J.*, 2, 108, 1988.
13. Kurt-Jones, E.A., Beller, D.I., Mizel, S.B., and Unanue, E.R., Identification of a membrane-associated interleukin-1 in macrophages, *Proc. Natl. Acad. Sci. U.S.A.*, 82, 1204, 1985.
14. Sims, J.E., Acres, R.B., Grubin, C.E., McMahan, C.J., Wignall, J.M., March, C.J., and Dower, S.K., Cloning the interleukin-1 receptor from human T cells, *Proc. Natl. Acad. Sci. U.S.A.*, 86, 8946, 1989.
15. McMahan, C.J., Slack, J.L., Mosley, B., Cosman, D., Lupton, S.D., Brunton, L.L., Grubin, C.E., Wignall, J.M., Jenkins, N.A., Branan, C.I., Copeland, N.G., Huebner, K., Croce, C.M., Cannizarro, L.A., Benjamin, D., Dower, S.K., Spriggs, M.K., and Sims, J.E., A novel IL-1 receptor, cloned from B cells by mammalian expression, is expressed in many cell types, *EMBO J.*, 10, 2821, 1991.

16. Hannum, C.H., Wilcox, C.J., Arend, W.P., Joslin, F.G., Dripps, D.J., Heimdal, P.L., Armes, L.G., Sommer, A., Eisenberg, S.P., and Thompson, R.C., Interleukin-1 receptor antagonist activity of a human interleukin-1 inhibitor, *Nature (London)*, 343, 336, 1990.
17. Gery, I., Gershon, R.K., and Waksman, B.H., Potentiation of the T lymphocyte response to mitogens. I. The responding cell, *J. Exp. Med.*, 136, 128, 1972.
18. Kaye, J., Gillis, S., Mizel, S.B., Shevach, E.M., Malek, T.R., Dinarello, C.A., Lachman, L.B., and Janeway, C.A., Jr., Growth of a cloned helper T cell line induced by a monoclonal antibody specific for the antigen receptor: interleukin-1 is required for the expression of receptors for interleukin-2, *J. Immunol.*, 133, 1339, 1984.
19. Gillis, S. and Mizel, S.B., T cell lymphoma model for the analysis of interleukin 1-mediated T-cell activation, *Proc. Natl. Acad. Sci. U.S.A.*, 78, 1133, 1981.
20. Gearing, A.J., Bird, C.R., Bristow, A., Poole, S., and Thorpe, R., A simple sensitive bioassay for interleukin-1 which is unresponsive to 10^3 units of interleukin-2, *J. Immunol. Methods*, 99, 7, 1987.
21. Schmidt, J.A., Mizel, S.B., Cohen, D., and Green, I., Interleukin 1, a potential regulator of fibroblast proliferation, *J. Immunol.*, 128, 2177, 1982.
22. Lachman, L.B., Brown, D.C., and Dinarello, C.A., Growth promoting effect of recombinant interleukin-1 and tumor necrosis factor for a human astrocytoma cell line, *J. Immunol.*, 138, 2913, 1987.
23. Kaye, J., Porcelli, S., Tite, J., Jones, B., and Janeway, C.A., Jr., Both a monoclonal antibody and antisera specific for determinants unique to cloned helper T cell lines can substitute for antigen and antigen-presenting cells in the activation of T cells, *J. Exp. Med.*, 158, 836, 1983.
24. Smith, K.A., Interleukin-2: inception, impact and implications, *Science*, 240, 1169, 1988.
25. Minami, Y., Kono, T., Miyazaki, T., and Taniguchi, T., The IL-2 receptor complex: its structure, function and target genes, *Annu. Rev. Immunol.*, 11, 245, 1993.
26. Russell, S.M., Keegan, A.D., Harada, N., Nakamura, Y., Noguchi, M., Leland, P., Friedmann, M.C., Miyajima, A., Puri, R.K., Paul, W.E., and Leonard, W.J., The interleukin-2 receptor γ chain is a functional component of the interleukin-4 receptor, *Science*, 262, 1880, 1993.
27. Kondo, M., Takeshita, T., Ishii, N., Nakamura, M., Watanabe, S., Arai, K., and Sugamura, K., Sharing of the interleukin-2 (IL-2) receptor γ chain between receptors for IL-2 and IL-4, *Science*, 262, 1874, 1993.
28. Noguchi, M., Nakamura, Y., Russell, S.M., Ziegler, S.F., Tsang, M., Cao, X., and Leonard, W.J., Interleukin-2 receptor γ chain: a functional component of the interleukin-7 receptor, *Science*, 262, 1877, 1993.
29. Zurawski, S.M., Vega, F., Jr., Huyghe, B., and Zurawski, G., Receptors for interleukin-13 and interleukin-4 are complex and share a novel component that functions in signal transduction, *EMBO J.*, 12, 2663, 1993.
30. Rubin, L.A. and Nelson, D.L., The soluble interleukin-2 receptor: biology, function and clinical application, *Ann. Intern. Med.*, 113, 619, 1990.
31. Bazill, G.W., Haynes, M., Garland, J., and Dexter, D.M., Characterization and partial purification of a hemopoietic growth factor in WEHI-3 conditioned medium, *Biochem. J.*, 210, 747, 1983.

32. Ben-Sasson, Z., Le Gros, G., Conrad, D.H., Finkelman, F., and Paul, W.E., Cross-linking Fc receptors stimulate splenic non-B non-T cells to secrete IL-4 and other lymphokines, *Proc. Natl. Acad., Sci., U.S.A.*, 87, 1421, 1990.
33. Schrader, J.W., The panspecific hemopoietin of activated T lymphocytes (interleukin-3), *Annu. Rev. Immunol.*, 4, 205, 1986.
34. Nicola, N.A., Hematopoietic cell growth factors and their receptors, *Annu. Rev. Biochem.*, 58, 45, 1990.
35. Nicola, N.A., and Metcalf, D., Subunit promiscuity among hemopoietic growth factor receptors, *Cell*, 67, 1, 1991.
36. Tavernier, J., Devos, R., Cornelis, S., Tuypens, T., Van der Heyden, J., Fiers, W., and Plaetnick, G., A human high affinity interleukin-5 receptor (IL-5R) is composed of an IL-5-specific α chain and a β chain shared with the receptor for GM-CSF, *Cell*, 66, 1175, 1991.
37. Dexter, T.M., Garland, J., Scott, P., Scolnick, E., and Metcalf, D., Growth of factor dependent hemopoietic precursor cell lines, *J. Exp. Med.*, 152, 1036, 1980.
38. Le Gros, G.S., Gillis, S., and Watson, J.D., Induction of IL-2 responsiveness in a murine IL-3-dependent T cell line, *J. Immunol.*, 139, 4009, 1985.
39. Greenberger, J.S., Sakakeeny, M.A., Humphries, R., Eaves, C., and Echner, R., Demonstration of a permanent factor-dependent multipotential hemopoietic progenitor cell lines, *Proc. Natl. Acad. Sci. U.S.A.*, 80, 2931, 1983.
40. Smith, C.A. and Rennick, D.M., Characterization of a murine lymphokine distinct from IL-2 and IL-3, possessing T cell growth factor activity and mast cell growth factor activity, *Proc. Natl. Acad. Sci. U.S.A.*, 83, 1857, 1986.
41. Kitamura, T., Tauge, T., Terasawa, T., Chiba, S., Kuwaki, T., Miyagawa, K., Piao, Y.-F., Miyazono, K., Urabe, A., and Takaku, F., Establishment and characterization of a unique human cell line that proliferates dependently on GM-CSF, IL-3 or erythropoietin, *J. Cell Physiol.*, 140, 323, 1989.
42. Le Gros, G.S., Le Gros, J.E., and Watson, J.D., The induction of lymphokine synthesis and cell growth in IL-3-dependent cell lines using antigen-antibody complexes, *J. Immunol.*, 139, 422, 1987.
43. Paul, W.E., Interleukin-4: a prototypic immunoregulatory lymphokine, *Blood*, 7, 1627, 1991.
44. Plaut, M., Pierce, J.H., Watson, D.J., Hanley-Hyde, J., Nordan, R.P., and Paul, W.E., Mast cell lines produce lymphokine in response to cross-linkage of FCεRI or to calcium ionophores, *Nature*, 339, 64, 1991.
45. Vitetta, E.S., Fernandez-Botran, R., Myers, C.D., and Sanders, V.M., Cellular interactions in the humoral immune response, *Adv. Immunol.*, 45, 1, 1989.
46. Finkelmann, F.D., Katona, I.M., Urban, J.F., Jr., Beckmann, M.P., Park, L.S., Schooley, K.A., Coffman, R.L., Mosmann, T.R., and Paul, W.E., Lymphokine control of *in vivo* immunoglobulin isotype selection, *Annu. Rev. Immunol.*, 8, 303, 1990.
47. Swain, S.L., Weinberg, A. D., English, M., and Huston, G., IL-4 directs the development of Th2-like helper effectors, *J. Immunol.*, 145, 3796, 1990.
48. Abeshira-Amar, O., Gilbert, M., Joliy, M., Theze, J., and Jankovic, D.L., IL-4 plays a dominant role in the differential development of Th0 into Th1 and Th2 cells, *J. Immunol.*, 148, 3820, 1992.
49. Seder, R.A., Paul, W.E., Davis, M.M., and de St. Groth, B.F., The presence of interleukin-4 during *in-vitro* priming determines the lymphokine producing potential of $CD4^+$ T cells from T cell receptor transgenic mice, *J. Exp. Med.*, 176, 1091, 1992.

50. Maher, D.W., Davis, I., Boyd, A.W., and Morstyn, G., Human interleukin-4: an immunomodulator with potential therapeutic applications, *Prog. Growth Factor Res.*, 3, 43, 1991.
51. Ohara, J. and Paul, W.E., Receptors for B-cell stimulatory factor-1 expressed on cells of hematopoietic lineage, *Nature*, 325, 537, 1987.
52. Park, L.S., Friend, D., Sassenfeld, H., and Urdal, D., Characterization of the high-affinity cell-surface receptor for murine B cell stimulating factor, *Proc. Natl. Acad. Sci. U.S.A.*, 84, 1669, 1987.
53. Lowenthal, J.W., Castle, B.E., Christiansen, J., Schreurs, J., Rennick, D., Arai, N., Hoy, P., Takebe, Y., and Howard, M., Expression of high-affinity receptors for murine interleukin-4 (BSF-1) on hemopoietic and nonhemopoietic cells, *J. Immunol.*, 140, 456, 1988.
54. Mosley, B., Beckman, M.P., March, C.J., Idzerda, R.L., Gimpel, S.D., VandenBos, T., Friend, D., Alpert, A., Anderson, J., Jackson, J., Wignall, J.M., Smith, C., Gallis, B., Sims, J.E., Urdal, D., Widmer, M.B., Cosman, D., and Park, L.S., The murine interleukin-4 receptor: molecular cloning and characterization of secreted and membrane bound forms, *Cell*, 59, 335, 1989.
55. Harada, N., Castle, B.E., Gorman, D.M., Itoh, N., Schreurs, J., Barrett, R.L., Howard, M., and Miyajima, A., Expression cloning of a cDNA encoding the murine interleukin 4 receptor based on ligand binding, *Proc. Natl. Acad. Sci. U.S.A.*, 87, 857, 1990.
56. Idzerda, R.L., March, C.J., Mosley, B., Lyman, S.D., Vandenbos, T., Gimpel, S.D., Din, W.S., Grabstein, K.H., Widmer, M.B., Park, L.S., Cosman, D., and Beckmann, M.P., Human interleukin 4 receptor confers biological responsiveness and defines a novel receptor superfamily, *J. Exp. Med.*, 171, 861, 1990.
57. Fernandez-Botran, R., and Vitetta, E.S., A soluble, high-affinity interleukin-4-binding protein is present in the biological fluids of mice, *Proc. Natl. Acad. Sci. U.S.A.*, 87, 4202, 1990.
58. Noelle, R., Krammer, P.H., Ohara, J., Uhr, J.W., and Vitetta, E.S., Increased expression of Ia antigens on resting B cells: an additional role for B cell growth factor, *Proc. Natl. Acad. Sci. U.S.A.*, 81, 6149, 1984.
59. Howard, M., Farrar, J., Hilfiker, M., Johnson, B., Takatsu, K., Hamaoka, T., and Paul, W.E., Identification of a T cell-derived B cell growth factor distinct from interleukin-2, *J. Exp. Med.*, 155, 914, 1982.
60. Vitetta, E.S., Ohara, J., Myers, C., Layton, J., Krammer, P.H., and Paul, W.E., Serological, biochemical and functional identity of B cell-stimulatory factor-1 and B cell differentiation factor for IgG1, *J. Exp. Med.*, 162, 1726, 1985.
61. Coffman, R.L. and Carty, J., A T cell activity that enhances polyclonal IgE production and its inhibition by interferon-γ, *J. Immunol.*, 136, 949, 1986.
62. Hu-Li, J., Ohara, J., Watson, C., Tsang, W., and Paul, W.E., Derivation of a T cell line that is highly responsive to IL-4 and IL-2 (CT.4R) and of an IL-2-hyporesponsive mutant of that line (CT.4S), *J. Immunol.*, 142, 800, 1989.
63. Idzerda, R.L., March, C.J., Mosley, B., Lyman, S.D., VandenBos, T., Gimpel, S.D., Din, W.S., Grabstein, K.H., Widmer, M.B., Park, L.S., Cosman, D., and Beckmann, M.P., Human interleukin-4 receptor confers biological responsiveness and defines a novel receptor superfamily, *J. Exp. Med.*, 171, 861, 1990.
64. Defrance, T., Vanbervliet, B., Aubry, J.P., Takebe, Y., Arai, N., Miyajima, A., Yokota, T., Lee, F., Arai, K., DeVries, J., and Banchereau, J., B cell growth-promoting activity of recombinant human interleukin-4, *J. Immunol.*, 139, 1135, 1987.

65. Rousset, F., de Waal Malefijt, R., Slierendregt, B., Aubry, J.P., Bonnefoy, J.Y., Defrance, T., Banchereau, J., and DeVries, J.E., Regulation of Fc-receptor for IgE (CD23) and class II MHC antigen expression of Burkitt's lymphoma cell lines by human interleukin-4, *J. Immunol.*, 140, 2625, 1988.
66. Sanderson, C.J., Warren, D.J., and Strath, M., Identification of a lymphokine that stimulates eosinophil differentiation *in vitro*. Its relationship to interleukin-3, and functional properties of eosinophils produced in cultures, *J. Exp. Med.*, 162, 60, 1985.
67. Campbell, H.D., Tucker, W.Q.J., Hort, Y., Martinson, M.E., Mayo, G., Clutterbuck, E.J., Sanderson, E.J., and Young, I.G., Molecular cloning, nucleotide sequence, and expression of the gene encoding human eosinophil differentiation factor (interleukin-5), *Proc. Natl. Acad. Sci. U.S.A.*, 84, 6629, 1987.
68. Swain, S.L., Howard, M., Kappler, J., Marrack, P., Watson, J., Booth, R., Wetzel, M., and Dutton, R.W., Evidence for two distinct classes of murine B cell growth factors with activities in different functional assays, *J. Exp. Med.*, 158, 822, 1983.
69. Brooks, K., Yuan, D., Uhr, J.W., Krammer, P.H., and Vitetta, E.S., Lymphokine-induced IgM secretion by clones of neoplastic B cells, *Nature (London)*, 302, 825, 1983.
70. Takatsu, K., Kikuchi, Y., Takahashi, T., Honjo, T., Matsumoto, M., Harada, N., Yamaguchi, N., and Tominaga, T., Interleukin-5, a T-cell-derived B-cell differentiation factor also induces cytotoxic T lymphocytes, *Proc. Natl. Acad. Sci. U.S.A.*, 84, 4234, 1987.
71. Swain, S.L. and Dutton, R.W., Production of a B cell growth-promoting activity, (DL)BCGF, from a cloned T cell line and its assay on the BCL_1 B cell tumor, *J. Exp., Med.*, 156, 1821, 1982.
72. Van Snick, J., Interleukin-6: an overview, *Annu. Rev. Immunol.*, 8, 253, 1990.
73. Kishimoto, T. and Hirano, T., Molecular regulation of B lymphocyte response, *Annu. Rev. Immunol.*, 6, 485, 1988.
74. Gearing, D.P., Comeau, M.R., Friend, D.J., Gimpel, S.D., Thut, C.J., McGourty, J., Brasher, K.K., King, J.A., Gillis, S., Mosley, B., Ziegler, S.F., and Cosman, D., The IL-6 signal transducer, gp130: an oncostatin M receptor and affinity converter for the LIF receptor, *Science*, 255, 1434, 1992.
75. Honda, M., Yamamoto, S., Chang, M., Yasukawa, K., Suzuki, H., Saito, T., Osugi, Y., Tokunaga, T., and Kishimoto, T., Human soluble IL-6-receptor: its detection and enhanced release by HIV infection, *J. Immunol.*, 148, 2175, 1992.
76. Aarden, L.A., De Groot, E.R., Schaap, O.L., and Lansdorp, P.M., Production of hybridoma growth factor by human monocytes, *Eur. J. Immunol.*, 17, 1411, 1987.
77. Van Snick, J., Cayphas, S., Vink, A., Uyttenhove, C., Coulie, P., and Simpson, R., Purification and NH_2-terminal amino acid sequence of a new T cell-derived lymphokine with growth factor activity for B cell hybridomas, *Proc. Natl. Acad. Sci. U.S.A.*, 83, 9679, 1986.
78. Namen, A.E., Schmierer, A.S., March, C.J., Overell, R.W., Park, L.S., Urdal, D.L., and Mochizuki, D.Y., B cell precursor growth promoting activity. Purification and characterization of a growth factor active on lymphocyte precursors, *J. Exp. Med.*, 167, 988,1988.

79. Goodwin, R.G., Lupton, S., Schmierer, A., Hjerrild, K.J., Jerzy, R., Clevenger, W., Gillis, S., Cosman, D., and Namen, A.E., Human interleukin-7: Molecular cloning and growth factor activity on human and murine B-lineage cells, *Proc. Natl. Acad. Sci. U.S.A.*, 86, 302, 1989.
80. Chazen, G.D., Pereira, G.M.B., Le Gros, G., Gillis, S., and Shevach, E.M., Interleukin-7 is a T cell growth factor, *Proc. Natl. Acad. Sci. U.S.A.*, 86, 5923, 1989.
81. Okazaki, H., Ito, M., Sudo, T., Hattori, M., Kano, S., Katsura, Y., and Minato, N., IL-7 promotes thymocytes bearing α/β or γ/δ T cell receptors *in vitro*: synergism with IL-2, *J. Immunol.*, 143, 2917, 1989.
82. Goodwin, R.G., Friend, D., Ziegler, S.F., Jerzy, R., Falk, B.A., Gimpel, S., Cosman, D., Dower, S., March, C.J., Namen, A.E., and Park, L.S., Cloning of the human and murine interleukin-7 receptors: demonstration of a soluble form and homology to a new receptor superfamily, *Cell*, 60, 941, 1990.
83. Park, L.S., Friend, D.J., Schmierer, A.S., Dower, S.K., and Namen, A.E., Murine interleukin 7 receptor. Characterization of an IL-7 dependent cell line, *J. Immunol.*, 171, 1073, 1990.
84. Whitlock, C.A. and Witte, O.N., Long-term culture of B lymphocytes and their precursors from murine bone marrow, *Proc. Natl. Acad. Sci. U.S.A.*, 79, 3608, 1982.
85. Ishihara, K., Median, K., Hayashi, S., Pietrangeli, C., Namen, A.E., Miyazaki, K., and Kincade, P.W., Stromal-cell and cytokine-dependent lymphocyte clones which span the pre-B to B-cell transition, *Devel. Immunol.*, 2, 149, 1991.
86. Van Snick, J., Goethals, A., Renauld, J.-C., Van Roost, E., Uyttenhove, C., Rubira, M.R., Moritz, R.L., and Simpson, R.J., Cloning and characterization of a cDNA for a new mouse T cell growth factor (P40), *J. Exp. Med.*, 169, 363, 1989.
87. Yang, Y.-C., Ricciardi, S., Ciarletta, A., Calvetti, J., Kelleher, K., and Clark, S.C., Expression cloning of a cDNA encoding a novel human hematopoietic growth factor: human homologue of murine T cell growth factor P40, *Blood*, 74, 1880, 1989.
88. Donahue, R.E., Yang, Y.-C., and Clark, S.C., Human P40 T cell growth factor (interleukin-9) supports erythroid colony formation, *Blood*, 75, 2271, 1990.
89. Moore, K.W., O'Garra, A., de Waal Maleyft, R., Vieira, P., and Mosmann, T.R., Interleukin-10, *Annu. Rev. Immunol.*, 11, 165, 1993.
90. Fiorentino, D.F., Bond, M.W., and Mosmann, T.R., Two types of mouse T helper cell. IV. Th2 clones secrete a factor that inhibits cytokine synthesis by Th1 clones, *J. Exp. Med.*, 170, 2081, 1989.
91. Moore, K.W., Vieira, P., Fiorentino, D.F., Trounstine, M.L., Khan, T.A., and Mosmann, T.R., Homology of cytokine synthesis inhibitory factor (IL-10) to the Epstein-Barr virus gene BCRFI, *Science*, 248, 1230, 1990.
92. Thompson-Snipes, L., Dhar, V., Bond, M.W., Mosmann, T.R., Moore, K.W., and Rennick, D., Interleukin 10: a novel stimulatory factor for mast cells and their progenitors, *J. Exp. Med.*, 173, 507, 1991.
93. Paul, S.R., Bennett, F., Calvetti, J.A., Kelleher, K., Wood, C.R., O'Hara, R.M., Leary, A.C., Sibley, B., Clark, S.C., Williams, D.A., and Yang, Y.-C., Molecular cloning of a cDNA encoding interleukin-11, a novel stromal cell-derived lymphopoietic and hematopoietic cytokine, *Proc. Natl. Acad. Sci. U.S.A.*, 87, 7512, 1990.

94. Quesniaux, V., Mayer, P., Liehl, E., Turner, K., Goldman, S., and Fagg, B., Review of a novel hematopoietic cytokine, interleukin-11, *Intl. Rev. Exp. Pathol.*, 34A, 205, 1993.
95. Yin, T., Miyazawa, K., and Yang, Y.-C., Characterization of interleukin-11 receptor and protein tyrosine phosphorylation induced by interleukin-11 in mouse 3T3-L1 cells, *J. Biol. Chem.*, 267, 8347, 1992.
96. Bennett, F., Giannotti, Clark, S.C., and Turner, K.J., Measurement of human interleukin-11, in *Current Protocols in Immunology,* Coligan, J.E., Kruisbeek, A.M., Margulies, D.H., Shevach, E.M., and Strober, W., Eds, Greene Publishing and Wiley InterScience, New York, 1991, 6.15.1.
97. Kobayashi, M., Fitz, L., Ryan, M., Hewick, R.M., Clark, S.C., Chan, S., Loudon, R., Sherman, F., Perussia, B., and Trinchieri, G., Identification and purification of a natural killer cell stimulatory factor (NKSF), a cytokine with multiple biological effects on human lymphocytes, *J. Exp. Med.*, 170, 827, 1989.
98. Stern, A.S., Podlaski, F.J., Hulmes, J.D., Pan, Y.-C.E., Quinn, P.M., Wolitzky, A.G., Familletti, P.C., Stremlo, D.L., Truitt, T., Chizzonite, R., and Gately, M.K., Purification to homogeneity and partial characterization of cytotoxic lymphocyte maturation factor from human B-lymphoblastoid cells, *Proc. Natl. Acad. Sci. U.S.A.*, 87, 6808, 1990.
99. Gately, M.K., Desai, B.B., Wolitzky, A.G., Quinn, P.M., Dwyer, C.M., Podlaski, F.J., Familletti, P.C., Sinigaglia, F., Chizzonite, R., Gubler, U., and Stern, A.S., Regulation of human lymphocyte proliferation by a heterodimeric cytokine, IL-12 (cytotoxic lymphocyte maturation factor), *J. Immunol.*, 147, 874, 1991.
100. Scott, P., IL-12: Initiation cytokine for cell-mediated immunity, *Science,* 260, 496, 1993.
101. Gately, M.K. and Chizzonite, R., Measurement of human and mouse interleukin-12, in *Current Protocols in Immunology,* Coligan, J.E., Kruisbeek, A.M., Margulies, D.H., Shevach, E.M., and Strober, W., Eds., Greene Publishing and Wiley InterScience, New York, 1991, 6.16.1.
102. Zurawski, G. and de Vries, J.E., Interleukin-13, an interleukin-4-like cytokine that acts on monocytes and B cells, but not T cells, *Immunol. Today,* 15, 19, 1994.
103. McKenzie, A.N.J., Culpepper, J.A., de Waal Maleyft, R., Briere, F., Punnonen, J., Aversa, G., Sato, A., Dang, W., Cocks, B.G., Menon, S., de Vries, J.E., Banchereau, J., and Zurawski, G., Interleukin-13, a novel T cell-derived cytokine that regulates human monocyte and B cell function, *Proc. Natl. Acad. Sci. U.S.A.*, 90, 3735, 1993.
104. de Waal Maleyft, R., Figdor, C., Huijbens, R., Mohan-Peterson, S., Bennet, B., Culpepper, J., Dang, W., Zurawski, G., and de Vries, J.E., Effects of IL-13 on phenotype, cytokine production, and cytotoxic function of human monocytes, *J. Immunol.*, 151, 6370, 1993.
105. Doherty, T.M., Kastelein, R., Menon, S., Andrade, S., and Coffman, R.L., Modulation of murine macrophage function by interleukin-13, *J. Immunol.*, 151, 7151, 1993.
106. McKenzie, A.N.J. and Zurawski, G., Measurement of interleukin-13, in *Current Protocols in Immunology,* Coligan, J.E., Kruisbeek, A.M., Margulies, D.H., Shevach, E.M., and Strober, W., Eds., Greene Publishing and Wiley InterScience, New York, 1991, 6.18.1.
107. Kundig, T.M., Schorle, H., Bachmann, M.F., Hengartner, H., Zinkernagel, R.M., and Horak, I., Immune responses in interleukin-2 deficient mice, *Science,* 262, 1059, 1993.

108. Center, D.N. and Cruishank, W., Modulation of lymphocyte migration by human lymphokines. I. Identification and characterization of chemoattractant activity for lymphocytes from mitogen-stimulated mononuclear cells, *J. Immunol.*, 128, 2563, 1982.
109. Cruishank, W., Berman, J.S., Theodore, A.C., Bernardo, J., and Center, D.N., Lymphokine activation of $T4^+$ lymphocytes and monocytes, *J. Immunol.*, 138, 3817, 1987.
110. Center, D.M., Kornfeld, H., and Cruishank, W.W., Interleukin 16 and its functions as a CD4 ligand, *Immunol. Today*, 17, 476, 1996.
111. Center, D.M., Cruishank, W.W., Parada, N.A., Ryan, T., Theodore, A.C., Viglianti, G., Lim, K.G., and Weller, P.F., Measurement of interleukin 16, in *Current Protocols in Immunology*, Coligan, J.E., Kruisbeek, A.M., Margulies, D.H., Shevach, E.M., and Strober, W., Eds., Greene Publishing and Wiley InterScience, New York, 1997, 6.23.1.
112. Fossiez, F., Djossou, O., Chomarat, P., Flores-romo, L., Ait-Yahia, S., Maat, C., Pin, J.-J., Garrone, P., Garcia, E., Saeland, S., Blanchard, D., Gaillard, C., Mahapatra, B.D., Rouvier, E., Goldstein, P., Banchereau, J., and Lebecque, S., T cell interleukin-17 induces stromal cells to produce proinflammatory and hematopoietic cytokines, *J. Exp. Med.*, 183, 2593, 1996.
113. Yao, Z., Painter, S.L., Fanslow, W.C., Ulrich, D., Macduff, B.M., Spriggs, M.K., and Armitage, R.J., Human IL-17: a new cytokine derived from T cells, *J. Immunol.*, 155, 5483, 1995.
114. Okamura, H., Tsutsui, H., Komatsu, T., Yutsudo, M., Hakura, A., Tanimoto, T., Torigoe, K., Okura, T., Nukada, Y., Hattori, K., Akita, K., Namba, M., Tanabe, F., Konishi, K., Fukuda, S., and Kurimoto, M., Cloning of a new cytokine that induces IFN-gamma production by T cells, *Nature (London)*, 378, 88, 1995.
115. Ushio, S., Namba, M., Okura, T., Hattori, K., Nukada, Y., Akita, K., Tanabe, F., Konishi, K., Micallef, M., Fujii, M., Torigoe, K., Tanimoto, T., Fukuda, S., Ikeda, M., Okamura, H., and Kurimoto, M., Cloning of the cDNA for human IFN-gamma-inducing factor, expression in *Escherichia coli*, and studies on the biologic activities of the protein, *J. Immunol.*, 156, 4274, 1996.
116. Tsutsui, H., Nakanishi, K., Matsui, K., Higashino, K., Okamura, H., Miyazawa, Y., and Kaneda, K., IFN-gamma-inducing factor up-regulates Fas ligand-mediated cytotoxic activity of murine natural killer cell clones, *J. Immunol.*, 157, 3967, 1996.
117. Yoshimoto, T., Okamura, H., Tagawa, Y., Iwakura, Y., and Nakanishi, K., Interleukin 18 together with interleukin 12 inhibits IgE production by induction of interferon-production from activated B cells, *Proc. Natl. Acad. Sci. U.S.A.*, 94, 3948, 1997.
118. Vassalli, P., The pathophysiology of tumor necrosis factors, *Annu. Rev. Immunol.*, 10, 411, 1992.
119. Carswell, E.A., Old, L.J., Kassel, R.L., Green, S., Fiore, N., and Williamson, B., An endotoxin-induced serum factor that causes necrosis of tumors, *Proc. Natl. Acad. Sci. U.S.A.*, 72, 3666, 1975.
120. Le, J. and Vilcek, J., Tumor necrosis factor and interleukin 1: cytokines with multiple overlapping biological activities, *Lab. Invest.*, 56, 234, 1987.

121. Engelmann, H., Aderka, D., Rubinstein, M., Rotman, D., and Wallach, D., A tumor necrosis factor-binding protein purified to homogeneity from human urine protects cells from tumor necrosis factor toxicity, *J. Biol. Chem.*, 264, 11974, 1989.
122. Seckinger, P., Isaaz, S., and Dayer, J.-M., Purification and biologic characterization of a specific tumor necrosis factor alpha inhibitor, *J. Biol. Chem.*, 264, 11966, 1989.
123. Gatanaga, T., Hwang, C.D., Kohr, W., Cappuccini, F., Lucci, J.A. III, Jeffes, E.W., Lentz, R., Tomich, J., Yamamoto, R.S., and Granger, G.A., Purification and characterization of an inhibitor (soluble tumor necrosis factor receptor) for tumor necrosis factor and lymphotoxin obtained from the serum ultrafiltrates of human cancer patients, *Proc. Natl. Acad. Sci. U.S.A.*, 87, 8781, 1990.
124. Hogan, M.M. and Vogel, S.N., Production of TNF by rIFN-γ-primed C3H/HeJ (Lps^d) macrophages requires the presence of lipid-A-associated proteins, *J. Immunol.*, 141, 4196, 1988.
125. Chen, A.R., McKinnon, K.P., and Koren, H.S., LPS stimulates fresh human monocytes to lyse actinomycin D-treated WEHI 164 target cells via increased secretion of a monokine similar to tumor necrosis factor, *J. Immunol.*, 135, 3979, 1985.
126. Pestka, S. and Baron, S., Definition and classification of the interferons, *Methods Enzymol.*, 78, 3, 1981.
127. Uze, G., Lutfalla, G., and Gresser, I., Genetic transfer of a functional human interferon α receptor into mouse cells: cloning and its expression of its cDNA, *Cell*, 60, 225, 1990.
128. Aguet, M., Dembic, Z., and Merlin, G., Molecular cloning and expression of the human interferon γ receptor, *Cell*, 55, 273, 1988.
129. Farrar, M.A. and Schreiber, R.D., The molecular cell biology of interferon-gamma and its receptor, *Annu. Rev. Immunol.*, 11, 571, 1993.
130. Rubinstein, S., Familletti, P.C., and Pestka, S., Convenient assay for interferons, *J. Virol.*, 37, 755, 1981.
131. King, D.P. and Jones, P.P., Induction of Ia and H-2 antigens on a macrophage cell line by murine interferon, *J. Immunol.*, 131, 315, 1983.
132. Schreiber, R.D., Hicks, L.J., Celada, A., Buchmeier, N.A., and Gray, P.W., Monoclonal antibodies to murine gamma interferon which differentially modulate macrophage activation and antiviral activity, *J. Immunol.*, 134, 1609, 1985.
133. Reynolds, D.S., Boom, W.H., and Abbas, A.K., Inhibition of B lymphocyte activation by interferon-γ, *J. Immunol.*, 139, 767, 1987.
134. Familletti, P.C., Rubinstein, and Pestka, S., A convenient and rapid cytopathic effect inhibition assay for interferon, *Methods Enzymol.*, 78, 387, 1981.
135. Schreiber, R.D., Measurement of mouse and human IFNγ, in *Current Protocols in Immunology*, Coligan, J.E., Kruisbeek, A.M., Margulies, D.H., Shevach, E.M., and Strober, W., Eds, Greene Publishing and Wiley InterScience, New York, 1991, 6.8.1.
136. Stanley, C.J., Johannsson, A., and Self, C.H., Enzyme amplification can enhance both the speed and the sensitivity of immunoassays, *J. Immunol. Methods*, 83, 89, 1985.

chapter seven

Chemokines

Contents

The chemokines are a family of chemotactic cytokines that signal through seven transmembrane receptors coupled to G_i-proteins.[1-3] Although originally identified and characterized based on their biological activity, many members of this family have been identified in the last few years through the application of bioinformatics and expressed sequence tag databases.[2] Approximately 40 or more chemokines have been identified to date. Chemokines have been classified into four families based on the expression of characteristic cysteine residues near their N-terminal end: CC-, CXC-, C-, and CX_3C, although a new standardized nomenclature has been proposed.[2] Nonetheless, the large number of chemokines has made it difficult to understand their individual relevance and physiological roles. Moreover, most chemokine receptors appear to have overlapping ligand specificities, contributing to the complexity of their study.[2,3]

As their name implies, the chemotactic function of chemokines was the first of their activities to be discovered and characterized.[1] Initially thought to be involved in directing the extravasation and migration of neutrophils and other cells of the innate immune system, it is now known that chemokines also attract different types and subsets of lymphocytes, and even some other types of cells. Moreover, chemokines have also been shown to participate in many other physiological processes, including angiogenesis/angiostasis, lymphoid traffic and lymphoid organ development, Th1/Th2 differentiation, wound healing, and metastasis.[1-3]

A thorough discussion of the different chemokines and their functions is beyond the scope of this chapter, and readers are urged to consult several excellent reviews available. Inasmuch as chemokines have many different functions and are active in a variety of systems, a wide variety of functional assays are available.[4] However, the chemotaxis assay remains the most widely functional assay for the identification and quantification of chemokines.[4,5] While the basic technique is fairly similar, the cell targets would vary depending on the chemokine being studied (e.g., neutrophils for IL-8, monocytes for MCP-1). In addition, other functional assays are also described. It is important to keep in mind that these functional assays are not chemokine-specific. Specific quantification of a chemokine in biological fluids, in which multiple chemokines are present, is normally done using an ELISA.

I. Microchemotaxis assay

Chemotaxis assays were routinely performed using single-well Boyden chambers, which made it difficult to analyze multiple samples.[4-6] The same assay has been modified to use multi-well chemotaxis chambers, allowing several samples to be investigated at one time.

Materials and reagents

- Recombinant human or murine chemokine standards (available commercially from a number of vendors, such as R & D Systems, BioSource, BD Pharmingen, Endogen)
- Chemotaxis medium: RPMI 1640 containing 25 m*M* HEPES and 0.5% fetal calf serum (heat inactivated) or 1% bovine serum albumin (without antibiotics or 2-mercaptoethanol)
- Multi-well Chemotaxis Chamber and accessories (Neuro Probe)
- Polycarbonate membranes with 3- to 5-μ*M* pores and with or without polyvinyl-pyrrolidone (PVP) coating (Neuro Probe)
- Extracellular matrix proteins: solutions of human plasma fibronectin, mouse collagen type I or IV, or mouse laminin (Gibco/BRL). Prepare at 20 μg/ml in H_2O.
- Cell suspension: Purified leukocyte or leukocyte subsets (Chapter 1)
- DiffQuik stain (Baxter, Muskegon, MI)
- Coverslips
- Glass slides
- Immersion oil
- Microscope
- Image analyzer (optional)

Protocol

1. Prepare serial dilutions of the sample to be analyzed in chemotaxis medium. Add in duplicates or triplicates to the bottom of wells in chemotaxis chamber (optimal volumes are approximately 25 to 28

μl/well). Take care not to overload the wells, as cross-contamination may occur. Alternatively, too small a volume will lead to the creation of bubbles that may interfere with cell migration.

2. Include a set of wells containing chemotaxis medium alone as a negative control. Set also positive controls (e.g., recombinant chemokines, see Table 7.1).

Table 7.1 Positive Controls for Cell Migration Assays

Cell Population	Chemokines/Reagents	Optimal Conc.
T lymphocytes	RANTES, MIP-1α, MIP-1β, MCP-1, MCP-2, MCP-3, lymphotactin	1–10 μ*M*
Monocytes, dendritic cells	RANTES, MIP-1α, MIP-1β, MCP-1, MCP-3, IP-10	3–30 μ*M*
Neutrophils	IL-8, MIP-2, NAP-2, ENA-78, GCP-2	3–30 μ*M*
	f-Met-Leu-Phe	10 n*M*

3. Place the polycarbonate membrane (shiny side up) over the filled wells of the chamber bottom. Quickly assemble the chamber gasket and lid, applying pressure on the chamber top until the assembly is secured in order to prevent cross-contamination.
4. The type of membrane used depends on the cells whose migration is being studied. Use PVP-coated filters for monocytes and dendritic cells and PVP-free filters for neutrophils and granulocytes. Optimal migration of lymphocytes is achieved using freshly prepared matrix-coated filters (prepared by floating the polycarbonate membrane in a 20-μg/ml solution of the matrix protein for 1 hr at 37°C or ovenight at 4°C, rinsing in PBS, and air-drying in a laminar flood hood).
5. Dilute the stock cell suspension to a cell density of 1×10^6 cells/ml in chemotaxis medium. Add 50 μl of the diluted cell suspension to the upper wells of the chemotaxis chamber. Incubate 1 to 4 hr at 37°C in a humidified air-CO_2 chamber.
6. Remove the assembly and decant the residual medium and cells. Gently scrape the original cell suspension-side of the membrane across wiper (provided by the manufacturer) to remove non-migrating cells. Repeat three to four times.
7. Hang membrane by clamp and air-dry for approximately 15 min. Stain filters in DiffQuik according to the manufacturer's directions. Mount filter on a slide, chemokine side up. Mark locations of the wells on the membrane with a marker. Add immersion oil and cover with a coverslip.
8. Count the cells. This can be done by eye under a 100X objective, or by image analysis. Results are expressed as the number of migrating

cells/5–10 high-power fields of membrane or as the percentage of migrating cells (relative to the total number).

9. The chemotactic index can be calculated as:

C.I. = Migrating cells to test reagent/Migrating cells in negative control

Comments

1. The activation state of the cell population may affect its chemotactic response. Generally, activation results in enhanced migratory response.
2. Migration times vary, depending on the cell population. Lymphocytes usually require longer incubation times (3 to 4 hr).
3. Cell migration can also be quantitated using fluorescently labeled cells, specially designed microplates, and a microfluorometer (NeuroProbe).
4. Different lots of matrix proteins may need to be tested for optimal activity.

II. Chemotaxis assay using Transwells

Chemotaxis assays can also be performed using Transwells (Costar, Cambridge, MA).[7] One advantage of this procedure is that it allows the determination of leukocyte migration through endothelial cells, which can be grown on top of the Transwell filters. Although considerable optimization needs to be done regarding the cell population under study and whether bare filter or endothelial cell-coated filters are used, the basic procedure is as given below.

Materials and reagents

- Recombinant human or murine chemokine standards (available commercially from a number of vendors, such as R & D Systems, BioSource, BD Pharmingen, Endogen)
- Chemotaxis medium: RPMI 1640 containing 25 m*M* HEPES and 0.5% fetal calf serum (heat inactivated) or 1% bovine serum albumin (without antibiotics or 2-mercaptoethanol)
- Transwell tissue-culture inserts/plates (6.5 mm diameter, 3 μm pore size) (Costar, Cambridge, MA; Cat. No. 3415)
- Cell suspension: purified leukocyte or leukocyte subsets (Chapter 1)
- Endothelial cell culture (e.g., HUVEC) in FK12 medium containing 10% FCS
- Incubator at 37°C and 5% CO_2
- Refrigerated centrifuge
- Pipettes
- Microscope

Protocol

1. For assays of cell migration through endothelial cell monolayers, harvest endothelial cells, count, and resuspend to a cell density of 2 $\times 10^6$ cell/ml in FK-12 medium containing 10% FCS. For assays using bare filters, skip to Step 5.
2. Add 600 µl of endothelial cell growth medium to the bottom wells of the Transwell plate.
3. Add 100 µl of the cell suspension to the Transwell inserts. Put the inserts on the bottom wells, making sure there are no bubbles under the filter.
4. Incubate the plates at 37°C in a humidified 5% CO_2 atmosphere for 24 to 48 hr to allow the monolayer to form.
5. Prepare serial dilutions of the sample to be analyzed and chemokine standards in chemotaxis medium. Assay in duplicates.
6. Add 600 µl of each dilution to the bottom wells. Include a negative control containing chemotaxis medium only. Place the plate in the incubator at 37°C while preparing the inserts so as to maintain the temperature.
7. Carefully remove the culture medium from the Transwell inserts, taking care not to touch the filter or disturb the cell monolayer.
8. Gently add 100 µl of the cell suspension (1×10^7 cells/ml in chemotaxis medium) to the Transwell inserts.
9. Place inserts in the bottom wells while trying to avoid trapping of air bubbles under the filters.
10. Transfer the plates to the incubator (37°C, 5% CO_2) and incubate for 1 to 3 hr.
11. After the incubation, remove the Transwell inserts from the plate and discard.
12. Resuspend the cells that have migrated into the bottom of the well.
13. Transfer an aliquot to a tube and count cells.

Comments

1. Counting of cells can be performed using light microscopy. Some endothelial cells may also be present and need to be distinguished from the migrating leukocytes.
2. Alternatively, the cells can be counted by flow cytometry or can be labeled with fluorescent dye and counted under a fluorescence microscope.

III. Other functional assays

Many other functional assays are available to study particular functions of chemokines on their target cells. Examples are calcium mobilization, actin polymerization, release of reactive oxygen intermediates, adherence to endothelial cells and extracellular matrix proteins.[4] Table 7.2 summarizes some of these functional assays, the target cells, and the chemokines that induce such responses.

Table 7.2 Functional Assays for Chemokines

Assay	Target Cells	Chemokines	Comments
Ca^{2+} mobilization	Monocytes, THP-1 cells	RANTES, MCP-1, MIP-1α	See Chapter 2
Reactive oxygen species release	Monocytes, neutrophils, eosinophils	RANTES, MCP-1, MIP-1α, IL-8, PAF, MCP-3, eotaxin, IL-5, IL-3	See Note 1
Actin polymerization	Neutrophils, eosinophils	RANTES, IL-8, PAF, eotaxin, IL-5	See Note 2
Histamine release[10]	Basophils, mast cells	RANTES, MCP-1, MCP-3, eotaxin, MIP-1α	
Adherence to endothelial cells/extracellular matrix proteins[3]	T lymphocytes	RANTES, MCP-1, MIP-1α	

Note:

1. Quantitated by superoxide anion (O^{2-}) production (superoxide dismutase inhibitable reduction of ferricytochrome C), staining of intracellular H_2O_2 with dihydrorhodamine 123 or lucigenin-dependent chemiluminiscence.[8]
2. Quantitated by staining of F-actin with 7-nitrobenz-2-oxa-1,3-diazol (NBD)-phallacidin and flow cytometry.[9]

References

1. Oppenheim, J.J., Zachariae, C.O.C., Mukaida, N., and Matsushima, K., Properties of the novel supergene "intercrine" cytokine family, *Annu. Rev. Immunol.*, 9, 817, 1991.
2. Sallusto, F., Mackay, C.R., and Lanzavecchia, A., The role of chemokine receptors in primary, effector, and memory immune responses, *Annu. Rev. Immunol.*, 18, 593, 2000.
3. Rossi, D. and Zlotnik, A., The biology of chemokines and their receptors, *Annu. Rev. Immunol.*, 18, 217, 2000.
4. Leonard, E.J., Sylvester, I., Yoshimura, T., Taub, D.D., Oppenheim, J.J., Wang, J.M., and Lloyd, A.R., Measurement of α and β chemokines, in *Current Protocols in Immunology,* Coligan, J.E., Kruiskeek, A.M., Margulies, D.H., Shevach, E.M., and Strober, W., Eds., Greene Publishing and Wiley InterScience, New York, 1995, 6.12.1.
5. Taub, D.D., Modified microchemotaxis assays, in *Methods in Molecular Biology, Vol. 138: Chemokine Protocols,* Proudfoot, A.E.I., Wells, T.N.C., and Power, C.A., Eds., Humana Press, Totowa, NJ, 2000, 105.

6. Harvath, L., Falk, W., and Leonard, E.J., Rapid quantitation of neutrophil chemotaxis: use of a polyvinylpyrrolidone-free polycarbonate membrane in a multiwell assembly, *J. Immunol. Methods*, 37, 39, 1980.
7. Donath, P.D., Wang, J., and Heath, H., Transwell chemotaxis, in *Methods in Molecular Biology, Vol. 138: Chemokine Protocols*, Proudfoot, A.E.I., Wells, T.N.C., and Power, C.A., Eds., Humana Press, Totowa, NJ, 2000, 113.
8. Elsner, J. and Kapp, A., Reactive Oxygen Release, in *Methods in Molecular Biology, Vol. 138: Chemokine Protocols*, Proudfoot, A.E.I., Wells, T.N.C., and Power, C.A., Eds., Humana Press, Totowa, NJ, 2000, 153.
9. Elsner, J. and Kapp, A., Actin polymerization, in *Methods in Molecular Biology, Vol. 138: Chemokine Protocols*, Proudfoot, A.E.I., Wells, T.N.C., and Power, C.A., Eds., Humana Press, Totowa, NJ, 2000, 149.
10. Lett-Brown, M.A. and Alam, R., Histamine release, Elsner, J. and Kapp, A., Reactive Oxygen Release, in *Methods in Molecular Biology, Vol. 138: Chemokine Protocols*, Proudfoot, A.E.I., Wells, T.N.C., and Power, C.A., Eds., Humana Press, Totowa, NJ, 2000, 157.

chapter eight

Cytokine receptors

Contents

I. Introduction

Cytokines exert their effects through binding to cytokine receptors expressed on the membrane of their target cells. In fact, the expression of cytokine receptors is one major mechanism regulating cytokine activity *in vivo*.[1,2] Initial attempts to characterize cytokine receptors by radioreceptor assays and receptor cross-linking studies yielded important information regarding receptor affinity and numbers, and the physical characteristics of cytokine-binding receptor components. However, it was not until recent years, with the development of anti-cytokine receptor monoclonal antibodies and the use of molecular techniques for the cloning and sequencing of the genes encoding cytokine receptors, that a much clearer picture of cytokine receptors and their mechanisms of function has emerged.[2,3]

In general, functional cytokine receptors are usually composed of two or more different subunits, with one or two subunits contributing the ligand-binding function and a different subunit functioning in signal-transduction.[3-8] It appears also that whereas the ligand-binding subunits alone have relatively low affinities for their ligands (low-affinity receptors), the interaction with the signal-transducing subunit stabilizes the binding, increasing the binding affinity several orders of magnitude (high-affinity receptors). Thus, these findings have provided an explanation for the previous observations of the heterogeneity of cytokine-binding sites (high- and low-affinity cytokine receptors) and that the biological activity was associated with the high-affinity receptors.[3-8]

Another observation that has found explanation in recent studies is that of the overlapping functions of obviously different cytokines. It is now evident that different cytokine receptors "share" common signal-transducing subunits, such as the case of the common γ_C-chain among IL-2R, IL-4R, IL-7R, IL-13R, and IL-15R;[3-6,9] and the β_C-chain shared among IL-3R, IL-5R, and GM-CSF-R.[7] Moreover, sequence homology comparisons have indicated that many cytokine receptors share common structural characteristics.[3,10] Based on these properties, cytokine receptors may belong to one of five different cytokine receptor families[11]:

1. The Class I or hemopoietin receptor family (including IL-2Rβ and γ chains, IL-4R, IL-5R, IL-7R, IL-9R, IL-12R, IL-13R, IL-15R, GM-CSFR and several hormone receptors)
2. The Class II or IFN receptor family (including IFNα/β-R and IFNγ-R)
3. The immunoglobulin superfamily (including IL-1R type I and II, IL-6R α-chain, IL-18R and M-CSFR)
4. The TNF receptor family (including TNF receptors type I and II, nerve growth factor receptor [NGF-R] and receptors for CD40 and Fas)
5. The seven-transmembrane helix family (including receptors for IL-8 and other chemokines)

A considerable understanding of the signaling mechanisms employed by different cytokine receptors has been achieved in recent years. For example, it is now known that Class I and II receptors function by associating with several JAK kinases, which are activated upon by ligand binding and receptor oligomerization. Downstream STAT transcription factors are then phosphorylated on tyrosine residues, inducing their dimerization and translocation into the nucleus where they bind to specific DNA sequences and regulate gene expression.[12,13] However, a thorough discussion on the signal transduction mechanisms of the different cytokine receptors is beyond the scope of this book.

Although membrane receptors have the obvious function of ligand binding and signal transduction, mounting evidence has indicated that many cytokine receptors also exist in soluble form.[1] These are truncated counterparts of the membrane receptors, generated either by "receptor shedding" or encoded by separate mRNAs that are released into biological fluids. The physiologic role of these soluble cytokine receptors (sCR) is not yet clear; however, because they retain their ligand-binding properties and inhibit binding of their respective ligands to membrane receptors, they are usually regarded as "cytokine antagonists."[1] Nonetheless, it has been demonstrated by several studies that sCR can, under some conditions, potentiate the activity of their ligands *in vivo*, probably as a result of increased half-life and/or altered biodistribution.[1,14,15] The functional role of sCR in immune responses and their potential use as prognostic "markers" remains to be studied further.

There are several approaches to the study of cytokine receptors, depending on the information sought. For example:

1. Radioreceptor assays, which measure binding of labeled cytokines to their receptors on target cells, give important information of receptor number and affinity(ies). These assays are very sensitive but usually require relatively large numbers of cells and adequate supply of cytokine (for labeling and competition studies).
2. Receptor cross-linking studies, which analyze the structure of cytokine-binding subunits by covalent cross-linking to the radiolabeled cytokine.
3. Flow cytometry, which detects cytokine receptor expression on cells based on reactivity with fluorochrome-labeled anti-receptor antibodies or cytokines. These assays require significantly lower number of cells than the radioreceptor assays, but their sensitivity is lower. Differences in the levels of receptor expression can be evaluated in a mixed-cell population.
4. Enzyme-linked immunoassays are the method of choice for the detection and quantitation of soluble cytokine receptors. The basic technique is the same as the one described for the cytokine ELISAs, with the only difference being that of the specific anti-cytokine antibodies. In addition, cellular ELISAs could also be adapted for the quantitation of membrane receptors.

A. Radioreceptor assay

The protocol described here allows the determination of receptor number and dissociation rate(s) based on Scatchard plots of equilibrium binding data.[16] The target cells are incubated in the presence of several concentrations of radiolabeled cytokine for a length of time sufficient to allow binding equilibrium to take place (~30 to 60 min). The amount of cytokine bound at each concentration is determined by centrifuging the cells through an oil gradient, allowing rapid separation of cell-bound from free cytokine, and then counting the cell pellets. Based on a plot of the amount of cytokine specifically bound vs. the ratio of bound/free cytokine at each concentration, it is possible to determine whether a homogeneous (straight line) or heterogeneous class of receptors exists (curvilinear line). In addition, receptor number and dissociation constant (Kd) can be estimated for each class of receptors. Readers are encouraged to familiarize themselves with the theoretical bases for these assays by consulting appropriate sources,[17,18] as they are not discussed in this chapter.

1. Binding assay

Materials and reagents

- Target cells (cell population to be assayed)
- Culture medium: RPMI-1640 containing 10% FCS
- PBS containing 1% FCS
- Radiolabeled cytokine, either labeled in the laboratory or purchased commercially (e.g., Amersham Pharmacia Biotech, NEN)
- Recombinant cytokine
- Dibutyl phthalate/dioctyl phthalate oil mixture (45/55) (Sigma)
- Microcentrifuge tubes (0.5- or 1.5-ml Eppendorf tubes)
- 400-μl microcentrifuge tubes with tips for collection of cell pellets (Sarstedt Cat. No. 72.702)
- 12 × 75-mm plastic tubes
- Ice bath
- Tabletop centrifuge, 4°C
- Microcentrifuge (Eppendorf)
- Large scissors or nail clippers
- γ-counter

Protocol

1. First determine the range and number of dilutions to be assayed. The range should be well below and above the dissociation rate (Kd). Because most cytokine receptors have Kd values in the range of 10 to 100 p*M*, a range covering from 0.5 p*M* to 10 n*M* should be attempted. Allow four tubes for each dilution. Two will receive the labeled cytokine only (for the estimation of total binding), and the other two will receive same concentration of labeled cytokine plus a 200-fold molar excess of unlabeled cytokine (for the estimation of nonspecific binding). Specific binding will then be calculated by subtraction of nonspecific from total binding at each concentration.
2. Binding reactions are performed in a final volume of 200 μl. Dilute the radiolabeled cytokine using culture medium and add 50 μl per tube. (Note that there will be a fourfold dilution once the cells and other reagents are added, so make dilutions accordingly.) Dilute the unlabeled cytokine stock and add 50 μl to each of the two tubes for the measurement of nonspecific binding, again taking into account the 1:4 dilution, or 50 μl of culture medium to the other two tubes measuring the total binding. Keep the tubes on an ice bath throughout the procedure.
3. Harvest the target cells and wash 3× with PBS-1% FCS by centrifugation at 200*g*. Count and resuspend the cells in culture medium to a density of 1×10^7 cells/ml. Using 1.5-ml Eppendorf tubes, add 100 μl of the cell suspension per tube (this will give a final cell number

of 1 × 10^6 cells per tube). Depending on the availability of cells and the relative number of receptors per cell, the number of cells per reaction can be varied from 0.5 to 5 × 10^6 cells per tube. Incubate on ice with gentle shaking until equilibrium is reached. The time to reach binding equilibrium needs to be determined in initial experiments, as it can vary from minutes to several hours.

4. While the Eppendorf tubes containing the cells and the labeled cytokine are being incubated, pipette 180 μl of the phthalate oil mixture into the same number of 400-μl microcentrifuge tubes. Spin the tubes briefly (1 to 2 sec) in an Eppendorf microcentrifuge (10,000 rpm) to release air bubbles trapped at the bottom of the tubes.
5. After equilibrium has been reached, load the contents of each Eppendorf tube on top of their respective oil-containing tubes. Centrifuge the 400-μl tubes in an Eppendorf microcentrifuge (10,000 rpm) for 20 sec. The cells should be pelleted at the bottom of the tips, whereas the medium should remain on top of the oil. With the aid of a large scissors or nail clippers, cut the tips of the tubes and place them in 12 × 75-mm plastic tubes. Care should be taken not to allow the oil to drip into these tubes.
6. Count the tips in a γ-counter. Also determine the total cpm added per tube by counting 20 μl of each labeled cytokine dilution.
7. For calculations, see section below.

Comments

1. See below for protocol for iodination (labeling) of cytokines.
2. When studying binding of a cytokine to cells that secrete it or that have been previously exposed to it (e.g., binding of IL-2 to HT-2 cells grown in IL-2-containing medium), cells must be first exposed to acid to remove any cytokine already bound to the membrane receptors. For this, first wash the cells in PBS-1% FCS to remove the free cytokine, then pellet the cells by centrifugation and resuspend the pellet for 30 sec in 1 to 2 ml culture medium adjusted to pH 3.0 with HCl. Quickly add the cells to 20 ml cold, regular culture medium and centrifuge. Wash the cells once and resuspend in culture medium at 4°C.

2. Iodination protocol

This protocol is based on the procedure described by Lowenthal et al.,[19] using Iodo-gen (Pierce)-coated tubes. The authors have used it with good results for the iodination of several cytokines, including rIL-4 and rIL-2. A number of alternative products for iodination are also available, such as Enzymobeads (Bio-Rad), Iodobeads (Pierce), and Bolton-Hunter reagent (Amersham Pharmacia Biotech, NEN). In addition, [^{125}I]-labeled human and mouse cytokines are also available from radioactive product vendors such as Amersham, Du Pont, ICN, etc.

Materials and reagents

- Iodo-gen™ (Pierce Cat. No. 28600)
- Recombinant cytokine (carrier-free)
- 1.5-ml Eppendorf tubes
- Iodine-125 (NaI-carrier free) (NEN, Cat. No. NEZ-033L)
- 0.2 *M* borate buffer, pH 8.5
- 0.2 *M* HEPES with 0.3 *M* NaCl, pH 5.35
- PBS-1% FCS
- Affinity column with antibody specific for cytokine
- Saline solution (0.15 *M* NaCl)
- Elution buffer: 50 m*M* citric acid, 0.15 *M* NaCl, pH 2.0
- 1 *M* Tris-HCl, pH 9.0
- Carrier protein: 10 mg/ml BSA in PBS
- Chloroform
- γ-counter
- Minicolumns (2 ml) (Bio-Rad)

Protocol

1. Prepare a 1 mg/ml solution of Iodo-gen in chloroform. Further dilute to 40 μg/ml by adding 40 μl of this solution to 960 μl of chloroform. Place 25 μl/tube of this solution into 1.5-ml Eppendorf tubes (1 μg Iodo-gen™ per tube). Evaporate the solvent under a gentle stream of nitrogen. Cap the tubes and store in the dark at room temperature. The tubes can be stored for several months.
2. Add 1 to 5 μg of recombinant cytokine in a volume of 25 μl buffer into the Iodo-gen-coated tube. Add approximately 1 mCi of iodine-125 diluted in 25 μl borate buffer, pH 8.5. Incubate on ice for 10 to 15 min.
3. Stop the reaction by transferring the contents to a clean Eppendorf tube. Add 50 μl of the HEPES-NaCl buffer and add to another Eppendorf tube containing approximately 1 ml of a 50% suspension of Sepharose beads coupled to the appropriate anti-cytokine monoclonal antibody in PBS-1% FCS.
4. Incubate for at least 1 hr at 4°C. Transfer the contents of the tube to a minicolumn (Bio-Rad) and wash beads with 15 × 1-ml aliquots of PBS-1% FCS, followed by 5 × 1-ml washes with saline. Monitor radioactivity.
5. Elute the bound material with 20 × 125-μl aliquots of elution buffer. Collect every two drops (~125 μl) into a separate tube containing 40 μl Tris-HCl (pH 9.0) and 10 μl BSA (10 mg/ml). Count radioactivity (it is best to take a 2-μl aliquot from each tube).

6. Plot cpm vs. fraction number. Pool those fractions within peak of radioactivity. Aliquot and store at –70°C.
7. Determine the concentration of bioactive cytokine in the labeled preparation by an appropriate bioassay (see Chapter 6).

Comments

1. The iodination protocol should be performed in a fumehood designated specifically for radioactive work. Follow appropriate precautions and safe handling of radioactive material.
2. Affinity chromatography is the most convenient way to remove free iodine. Alternatively, this separation could also be accomplished by gel filtration using a 1-ml column of Sephadex G-25. The affinity column medium can be prepared by coupling the appropriate anti-cytokine monoclonal antibody to Affi-gel 10 beads (Bio-Rad) following the manufacturer's instructions.
3. Labeled cytokines should be stored in the presence of a carrier protein.

3. Calculations

Scatchard plots of equilibrium binding data (concentration of bound ligand on the *x*-axis vs. ratio of bound/free ligand at each concentration tested on the *y*-axis) provide important information on several parameters, including:

- Presence of a single or multiple classes of binding sites (e.g., high- and low-affinity receptors) (Scatchard plots yielding a straight line are indicative of a single affinity, whereas a curved line may mean receptors of two or more different affinities and/or negative co-operativity).
- Dissociation constant(s) (Kd), given by the reciprocal of the slope of the curve(s)
- Number of binding sites (Bmax), given by the intercept of the line at the *x*-axis

These parameters can be calculated manually or, alternatively, with the aid of a number of computer programs for analysis of binding data.[20] These programs will calculate the best fit for the curves and provide information about the classes and number of binding sites and their dissociation constants.

1. For calculation, create a table with the following columns:
   a. The concentrations of [^{125}I]cytokine tested (in molar units)
   b. Total cpm bound at each concentration
   c. Nonspecific binding at each concentration (cpm)

2. Calculate the specific binding at each concentration by subtracting nonspecific binding (column **c**) from total binding (column **b**). Nonspecific binding should be linear. Place results in column (**d**).
3. Write the total cpm added at each concentration in column (**e**). Now calculate the concentration of bound ligand by dividing the values in column (**d**) (specific binding, in cpm) by the total cpm values (in column **e**) and multiplying the result by the ligand concentration (in column **a**). Write the result in column (**f**); this is the concentration of bound ligand in molar units.

$$[\text{Bound ligand}]\ (\mathbf{f}) = (\mathbf{d}/\mathbf{e}) \times \mathbf{a}$$

4. Calculate the free ligand concentration by subtracting the bound ligand concentration in column (**f**) from initial ligand concentration in column (**a**). Place the result in column (**g**).
5. Calculate the ratio of bound/free ligand by dividing the bound ligand concentration in column (**f**) by the free ligand concentration of column (**g**). Place the result in column (**h**). All the concentration values are in molar units.
6. Plot the bound ligand concentration, in column (**f**) on the x-axis vs. the bound/free ratio in column (**h**).
7. Calculate the best-fitting curve. If the resulting curve is a straight line (which can be fitted by simple linear regression analysis), this indicates a single affinity. The apparent dissociation constant is given by the reciprocal of the slope of the curve. Its values are in molar units. If the resulting curve is not straight, indicative of receptors of more than one affinity, the data can be resolved into two different affinity components (high and low affinity), which are plotted and analyzed separately, treating each component as a single class of receptors.

$$\text{Dissociation constant (Kd)} = 1/\text{Slope (in molar units)}$$

8. From the linear regression analysis: $y = mx + b$, where "m" is the slope and "b" is the intercept at the y-axis. To calculate the number of receptors per cell, first calculate the intercept at the x-axis (maximal amount of ligand bound) by dividing the intercept at y (b) by the slope (m). The result (in molar units) is then multiplied by the assay volume in liters (2×10^{-4}), multiplied by 6.02×10^{23} molecules/mole (Avogadro's number) and divided by the number of cells used in each tube (e.g., 1×10^{6} cells). Assuming that each receptor binds one single molecule of ligand, the resulting number should equal the number of receptors per cell.

$$\text{No. of receptors/cell} = (b \div m) \times \text{Vol. in liters} \times 6.02 \times 10^{23} \times 1/\text{No. of cells}$$

B. Cross-linking of labeled cytokines to their receptors

Important information regarding the composition of high- and low-affinity receptors and the molecular weight of receptor subunits can be obtained by the covalent cross-linking of an iodinated cytokine to its membrane receptors, followed by SDS-PAGE analysis of the cell lysate. Although a wide variety of homofunctional and heterofunctional cross-linking reagents are available (Pierce, Rockford, IL), two of the most commonly used in cytokine receptor analysis are disuccinimidyl suberate (DSS) and dithio-bis(succinimidyl propionate) [DSP].[21-23] Cross-linking by DSS is irreversible, whereas cross-linking by DSP is reversible by sulfhydryl reagents. The basic protocol is similar.

Materials and reagents

- Target cells
- Culture medium: RPMI containing 10% FCS
- PBS-1% FCS
- PBS
- [^{125}I]-labeled cytokine (see this chapter, Section A)
- Disuccinimidyl suberate (DSS; Pierce Cat. No. 21555 G) or dithio-bis(succinimidyl propionate) (DSP; Pierce Cat. No. 22585G)
- Dimethylsulfoxide (DMSO)
- PBS-containing 20 m*M* L-lysine, pH 7.25
- Lysis buffer: PBS containing 1% NP 40, 1 m*M* phenylmethylsulfonyl fluoride and 1 m*M* EDTA, pH 7.25 (Sigma)
- Reagents and equipment necessary for SDS-PAGE analysis and autoradiography
- Centrifuge tubes (15 and 50 ml)
- Eppendorf microcentrifuge tubes (1.5 ml)
- Refrigerated centrifuge
- Ice bath

Protocol

1. Harvest the target cells. Wash the cells 3× in cold PBS-1% FCS. Count and resuspend at 1×10^7 cells/ml in culture medium (15-ml centrifuge tube). Place the tube on ice.
2. Add the radiolabeled cytokine to the desired concentration. Most high-affinity cytokine receptors will be occupied if the ligand concentration is approximately 1 to 2×10^{-10} *M*. However, for binding to low-affinity

receptors, higher concentrations of ligand (~1 to 2 × 10^{-9}) are required. Incubate for 60 min on ice with occasional shaking.

3. Wash the cells once in 15 ml ice-cold PBS and aspirate the supernatant. Resuspend cell pellet in 0.5 ml cold PBS.
4. Dissolve DSP in DMSO to a final concentration of 100 m*M*. Make a 1:100 dilution by taking 10 µl of this solution and adding it to 990 µl cold PBS, while vortexing. Add 0.5 ml diluted DSP solution to the cell suspension. (The final DSP concentration is 0.5 m*M*, and the final DMSO concentration is 0.5%.) For DSS, use a 1:40 dilution of a 100 m*M* DSS solution in DMSO (final concentration of DSS is 2 m*M*). Incubate for 30 min on ice with occasional shaking.
5. Inactivate and remove the cross-linker by washing once with 13 ml cold PBS containing L-lysine and twice with PBS-1% FCS.
6. Aspirate the last wash and resuspend the cell pellet in ~150 µl of lysis buffer. Incubate for 15 min on ice.
7. Transfer the lysate to a 1.5-ml microcentrifuge tube and centrifuge in an Eppendorf centrifuge (~10,000 rpm) for 5 min to separate nuclei and insoluble debris.
8. At this point, the supernatants can be mixed with an equal volume of 2X SDS-PAGE sample buffer and electrophoresed directly, or the lysates can be first immunoprecipitated with the appropriate anti-cytokine receptor antibodies and then analyzed by SDS-PAGE.
9. After electrophoresis, fix the gels with 40% methanol containing 10% trichloroacetic acid, dry the gel, and visualize bands by autoradiography.

Comments

1. Incubation of cells with ligand at 4°C prevents internalization of the receptor.
2. It is recommended to include specificity controls, in which the cells are incubated with the iodinated cytokine in the presence of a 100-fold molar excess of unlabeled cytokine. In addition, other controls should include:
   a. Cells plus labeled cytokine without cross-linking reagent
   b. Labeled cytokine alone plus cross-linking reagent
3. The cross-linking reagent must be prepared fresh just prior to use.
4. Samples cross-linked with DSS can be analyzed by SDS-PAGE under both reducing and nonreducing conditions. Samples cross-linked with DSP can be analyzed only under nonreducing conditions, as reducing agents cleave the cross-linker.

C. *Analysis of cytokine receptors by flow cytometry*

The relative expression of cytokine receptors (or cytokine receptor subunits) can also be analyzed by flow cytometry after staining of target cells with appropriate fluorochrome-conjugated anti-cytokine receptor antibodies or cytokines. The advantages of this technique are that relatively small numbers of cells are needed and that no radioactive reagents are required. This method, however, is less sensitive and quantitative than the radioreceptor-binding assay (cells expressing only a few hundred receptors per cell may not stain very brightly). Anti-cytokine receptor antibodies (both human and murine) are available from several sources and can be used directly labeled with FITC (or other fluorochrome) or coupled to a biotin-avidin-FITC detection system. (The protocols used for staining and analysis were described in Chapter 2.)

In addition, both human and mouse cytokines coupled to FITC can be purchased from R & D Systems.

D. ELISA for detection of soluble cytokine receptors

Detection and quantification of soluble cytokine receptors in tissue culture supernatants or biological fluids are usually performed by the same sandwich-ELISA method as described in Chapters 6 and 9. The protocols for plate coating, capture, and detection are identical, with exception of the appropriate anti-cytokine receptor antibodies. One important point to take into consideration when assaying soluble cytokine receptors is the fact that the binding of anti-receptor antibodies may be blocked by the presence of endogenously secreted receptor ligand (cytokine). For example, the authors have determined that the reactivity of the murine soluble IL-4 receptor with M1, an anti-IL-4R monoclonal antibody is inhibited by the presence of IL-4. One approach to avoid interference by endogenously secreted IL-4 in this case is to preincubate the samples with an excess of a neutralizing anti-IL-4 monoclonal antibody (10 μg/ml) for 60 min at 37°C and then perform the sIL-4R capture and detection.

Alternatively, detection of captured soluble cytokine receptors has been accomplished by binding of a radiolabeled cytokine preparation instead of a second anti-receptor monoclonal antibody. In this case, however, the capture antibody must not prevent ligand binding.

For soluble receptors with potential clinical diagnostic or prognostic applications, such as soluble IL-2R and soluble TNF-R, ELISA kits have been developed and can be purchased from different vendors, including AMAC, Immunotech, T Cell Diagnostics, and Biosource.

References

1. Fernandez-Botran, R., Soluble cytokine receptors: their role in immunoregulation, *FASEB J.*, 5, 2567, 1991.
2. Taga, T. and Kishimoto, T., Cytokine receptors and signal transduction, *FASEB J.*, 7, 3387, 1993.
3. Boulay, J.L. and Paul, W.E., The interleukin-4-related lymphokines and their binding to hemopoietin receptors, *J. Biol. Chem.*, 267, 20525, 1992.

4. Kondo, M., Takeshita, T., Ishii, N., Nakamura, M., Watanabe, S., Arai, K., and Sugamura, K., Sharing of the interleukin-2 (IL-2) receptor γ chain between receptors for IL-2 and IL-4, *Science*, 262, 1874, 1993.
5. Noguchi, M., Nakamura, Y., Russell, S.M., Ziegler, S.F., Tsang, M., Cao, X., and Leonard, W.J., Interleukin-2 receptor γ chain: a functional component of the interleukin-7 receptor, *Science*, 262, 1877, 1993.
6. Zurawski, S.M., Vega, F., Jr., Huyghe, B., and Zurawski, G., Receptors for interleukin-13 and interleukin-4 are complex and share a novel component that functions in signal transduction, *EMBO J.*, 12, 2663, 1993.
7. Nicola, N.A. and Metcalf, D., Subunit promiscuity among hemopoietic growth factor receptors, *Cell*, 67, 1, 1991.
8. Gearing, D.P., Comeau, M.R., Friend, D.J., Gimpel, S.D., Thut, C.J., McGourty, J., Brasher, K.K., King, J.A., Gillis, S., Mosley, B., Ziegler, S.F., and Cosman, D., The IL-6 signal transducer, gp130: an oncostatin M receptor and affinity converter for the LIF receptor, *Science*, 255, 1434, 1992.
9. Grabstein, K.H., Eisenman, J., Shanebeck, K., Rauch, C., Srinivasan, S., Fung, V., Beers, C., Richardson, J., Schoenborn, M.A., Ahdieh, M., Johnson, L., Alderson, M.R., Watson, J.D., Anderson, D.M., and Giri, J.G., Cloning of a T cell growth factor that interacts with the β chain of the interleukin-2 receptor, *Science*, 264, 965, 1994.
10. Bazan, J.F., A novel family of growth factor receptors: a common binding domain in the growth hormone, prolactin, erythropoietin and IL-6 receptors, and the p75 IL-2 receptor β-chain, *Biochem. Biophys. Res. Commun.*, 164, 788, 1989.
11. Abbas, A.K., Lichtman, A.H., and Pober, J.S., *Cellular and Molecular Immunology*, 2nd. ed., Saunders, Philadelphia, 1994, 240.
12. Ihle, J.N., Witthuhn, B.A., Quelle, F.W., Yamamoto, K., and Silvennoinen, O., Signaling through the hematopoietic cytokine receptors, *Annu. Rev. Immunol.*, 13, 369, 1995.
13. Bach, E.A., Aguet, M., and Schreiber, R.D., The IFN gamma receptor: a paradigm for cytokine receptor signaling, *Annu. Rev. Immunol.*, 15, 369, 1997.
14. Sato, T.A., Widmer, M.B., Finkelman, F.D., Madani, H., Jacobs, C.A., Grabstein, K.H., and Maliszewski, C.R., Recombinant soluble murine IL-4 receptor can inhibit or enhance IgE responses *in vivo*, *J. Immunol*, 150, 2717, 1993.
15. Finkelman, F.D., Madden, K.B., Morris, S.C., Holmes, J.M., Katona, I.M., and Maliszewski, C.R., Anticytokine antibodies as carrier proteins: prolongation of *in vivo* effects of exogenous cytokines by injection of cytokine-anti-cytokine antibody complexes, *J. Immunol.*, 151, 1235, 1993.
16. Scatchard, G., The attractions of proteins for small molecules and ions, *Ann. N.Y. Acad. Sci.*, 51, 660, 1949.
17. Weiland, G.A. and Molinoff, P.B., Quantitative analysis of drug-receptor interactions: I. Determination of kinetic and equilibrium properties, *Life Sciences*, 29, 313, 1981.
18. Molinoff, P.B., Wolfe, B.B., and Weiland, G.A., Quantitative analysis of drug-receptor interactions. III. Determination of the properties of receptor subtypes, *Life Sciences*, 29, 427, 1981.
19. Lowenthal, J.W., Castle, B.E., Christiansen, J., Schreurs, J., Rennick, D., Arai, N., Hoy, P., Takebe, Y., and Howard, M., Expression of high-affinity receptors for murine interleukin-4 (BSF-1) on hemopoietic and nonhemopoietic cells, *J. Immunol.*,140, 456, 1988.

20. Munson, P.J., LIGAND: a computerized analysis of ligand binding data, *Methods Enzymol.*, 92, 543, 1983.
21. Sharon, M., Klausner, R.D., Cullens, B.R., Chizzonite, R., and Leonard, W.J., Novel interleukin-2 receptor subunit detected by cross-linking under high affinity conditions, *Science*, 234, 859, 1986.
22. Saragovi, H. and Malek, T.R., The murine interleukin 2 receptor: irreversible cross-linking of radiolabeled interleukin 2 to high affinity interleukin 2 receptors reveals a noncovalently associated subunit, *J. Immunol.*, 139, 1918, 1987.
23. Fernandez-Botran, R., Sanders, V.M., and Vitetta, E.S., Interactions between receptors for interleukin 2 and interleukin 4 on lines of helper T cells (HT-2) and B lymphoma cells (BCL_1), *J. Exp. Med.*, 169, 379, 1989.

chapter nine

Antibodies

Contents

I. Polyclonal antibodies

The choice of animal for antibody production depends primarily upon the amount of anti-serum desired. The two most common choices are mice and rabbits. The experimental protocol for successful immunization depends significantly on the type and immunogenicity of an antigen. Therefore, only general points of consideration can be provided here.

The protein antigen is injected intradermally, intramuscularly, or subcutaneously in the presence of adjuvant. At least four different types of adjuvant are commonly used: (1) complete Freund's adjuvant (Sigma), (2) MPL and TDM Emulsion (Ribi Immunochem Research, Inc.), (3) TiterMax (CytRx Corp.), or (4) Gerbu adjuvant (Biotech). The latter three offer significantly higher titers and, in some cases, even easier handling. On the negative side, their price is significantly higher than that of complete Freund's adjuvant.

Always remember to collect a sample of serum prior to immunization (as a negative control for future tests). In general, booster immunizations should start 4 to 8 weeks after the first injection and should continue at 3-week intervals. For most soluble protein antigens, specific antibodies begin to appear in the blood 5 to 8 days after immunization.

The alternative to the use of an adjuvant or a method for increasing the immunogenicity is to couple the protein antigens to a carrier protein. The two most commonly used carriers are keyhole limpet hemocyanine (KLH) and bovine serum albumin (BSA).

A. Preparation of complete Freund's adjuvant-antigen emulsion

Materials and reagents

- Complete Freund's adjuvant (CFA; Sigma)
- Antigen
- 3-ml glass syringes
- Double-ended locking hub connector
- 21-G needle

Protocol

1. Shake the bottle with CFA well to disperse insoluble *Mycobacterium tuberculosis* bacilli.
2. Mix 2 ml CFA with 2 ml of a 2 mg/ml solution of antigen.
3. Draw this mixture up into a 3-ml glass syringe. Attach a double-ended locking hub connector already connected to an empty 3-ml glass syringe. Repeatedly force the mixture back and forth from one syringe to the other. When the mixture is white and quite homogenous, remove the connector and attach a 21-G needle.
4. Remove all air bubbles and inject CFA-antigen emulsion into multiple sites in the animal.

Comments

1. The volumes shown above can be scaled down according to individual needs. The use of proportionally smaller syringes will be advantageous.
2. CFA is extremely inflammatory. Always use gloves and protective eyewear.
3. For booster immunization, use incomplete Freund's adjuvant (Sigma) instead of CFA.
4. To determine whether the solution is homogeneous, put a small drop of antigen-adjuvant mixture onto the surface of 50 ml cold water in a beaker. If the drop disperses, continue mixing the antigen as described in Step 3.

B. *Ribi adjuvant*

This adjuvant consists of purified microbial components in a metabolizable oil. While a combination of monophosphoryl lipid A and synthetic trehalose dicorynomycolate is optimal for the use with strong immunogens, synthetic trehalose dicorynomycolate alone is preferred for regular-strength immunogens.

Materials and reagents

- Ribi adjuvant (Ribi Immunochem Research, Inc.)
- Water bath
- Syringe
- 21-G needle
- Saline
- Antigen
- Vortex

Protocol

1. Warm the vial to 45°C for 10 min. Inject 2 ml saline with desired amount of antigen directly into the vial through the rubber stopper. Vortex vigorously for 3 min.
2. Immunize mice with 0.1 ml subcutaneously in two sites or 0.2 ml intraperitoneally. For rats and guinea pigs, inject 0.2 ml subcutaneously in two sites and 0.1 ml intraperitoneally.
3. Repeat on day 21 and test bleed 1 week later. If necessary, repeat the injection every 21 days.

Comments

1. Recommended antigen concentration is from 0.05 to 0.25 mg/ml in saline.
2. For larger animals (goats, sheep, pigs, and rabbits), use a cell wall skeleton, monophosphoryl lipid A, and synthetic trehalose dicorynomycolate mixture.
3. Stability of water-in-oil emulsion can be checked by placing a drop of emulsion on water. The emulsion should hold together.

C. *TiterMax adjuvant*

The adjuvant contains a synthetic polymer CRL-8941 composed of chains of hydrophobic polyoxypropylene and hydrophilic polyoxyethylene. In addition, microparticulate silica coated with CRL-8941, sorbitan monooleate 80, and squalene are also present. As the adjuvant contains no protein or peptide, there is no toxicity. Squalene is a completely metamolizable oil. A comparison of commercially available adjuvants showed that TiterMax induced higher and longer-lasting titers with fewer injections than with any other adjuvant.[1] In addition, the inflammatory responses were milder and more transient.

Materials and reagents

- TiterMax (CytRx Corp.)
- Antigen
- 18-G needle
- 3-ml plastic syringes
- 18-G double-hub emulsification needle
- Vortex

Protocol

1. Warm the TiterMax to room temperature and vortex for 30 sec.
2. Load a syringe with appropriate volume of TiterMax.

3. Load the second syringe with half the amount of antigen in aqueous medium.
4. Connect the two syringes via a double-hub emulsification needle and mix the material by forcing it back and forth through the needle for 1 min. The formation of a water-in-oil emulsion is signaled by a sudden increase in viscosity.
5. Push all of the emulsion into one syringe, disconnect the empty syringe, and load the empty syringe with the remaining antigen.
6. Reconnect the syringes and emulsify for another 30 to 60 seconds.

Comments

1. It is important to add the aqueous antigen to the TiterMax in at least two volumes.
2. It is important to push the antigen into the TiterMax syringe first.
3. The stability of the water-in-oil emulsion can be checked by placing a drop of emulsion on water. The emulsion should hold together.
4. The syringes should be all plastic, as rubber pistons contain a lubricant that fails in the presence of TiterMax and causes the syringes to stick.

II. Monoclonal antibodies

The use of monoclonal antibodies has proliferated more than almost any other immunological technique. Monoclonal antibodies, for example, are widely used in cell biology, biochemistry, pathology, oncology, hematology, physiology, molecular genetics, and microbiology. The idea of immortalization of specific antibody-forming cells by their fusion with myeloma cells was first introduced by Köhler and Milstein.[2] Since then, numerous modifications have been published but all are only variations of the original technique.[3-6]

The idea is basically quite simple. The partner tumor cell line is resistant to the purine analogue 6-thioguanine due to its deficiency of hypoxanthine-guanine phosphoribosyl transferase. The result of this deficiency is a high sensitivity to aminopterine. Normal B lymphocytes are resistant to aminopterine in the presence of hypoxanthine and thymidine (they utilize salvage pathways). While the B cell causes an immortality of the fused cells in HAT medium, the tumor cell causes the immortality in all subsequent feedings.

Materials and reagents

- DME/F12 HYBRI-MAX medium (Sigma) with sodium pyruvate, amino acids, antibiotics, and 10% FCS (for P653 cells) or 20% FCS
- DME/F12 HYBRI-MAX medium without FCS (Sigma)
- HAT (Sigma): 1 ml of 50X concentrated powder (diluted in 10 ml medium without FCS) per 50 ml of medium with 20% FCS + 20% CM

- HT (Sigma): 1 ml of 50X concentrated powder (diluted in 10 ml medium without FCS) per 50 ml of medium with 20% FCS + 20% CM
- Conditioned medium (CM) (i.e., supernatant from P653 cells)
- Sterile water
- Polyethylene glycol (PEG) 1500 (Boehringer-Mannheim, Sigma
- Immunized mice (boosted with antigen 3 days prior to harvesting)
- 96-well tissue culture plates (Costar)
- 6-well tissue culture plates (Costar)
- 24-well tissue culture plates (Costar)
- P3 X63-Ag8.653 cells (P653; ATCC)
- 50-ml conical centrifuge tubes
- 1-ml pipettes
- 10-ml pipettes
- Humidified, 5% CO_2 incubator
- Glass beakers

Protocol

(*Note*: All materials and reagents must be sterile and proper aseptic techniques must be used when handling the cells.)

1. Split P653 cells 24 hr before fusion and cultivate in DME/F12 HYBRI-MAX medium with 10% FCS.
2. Store conditioned medium.
3. Wash P653 cells 3× with serum-free medium by centrifugation at 500 × *g* for 5 min at room temperature and count them.
4. Sacrifice mice and store the serum from the mice. It will be used as a positive control for later screening.
5. Prepare a spleen cell suspension and place the cells into 50-ml centrifuge tubes. Wash once with serum-free medium by centrifugation at 500*g* for 10 min at room temperature.
6. Lyse the erythrocytes by pouring 2 ml sterile water on the pellet. Count to 20, fill with serum-free medium, and immediately spin. Discard supernatant and add 45 ml serum-free medium. Centrifuge (500*g* for 5 min at room temperature) again. Wash 3× with serum-free medium under the same conditions. Resuspend spleen cells in serum-free medium and count them.
7. Mix P653 myeloma cells and spleen cells at a 1:10 ratio in a 50-ml centrifuge tube and fill the tube with serum-free medium. Centrifuge at 500*g* for 5 min at room temperature.
8. Prewarm PEG solution to 37°C.
9. Prewarm 20 ml serum-free medium to 37°C.
10. Discard supernatant from the cell mixture (Step 7).
11. Put the centrifuge tube with the cell mixture into a 37°C water bath (place a beaker with warm water into the hood). Using a 1-ml pipette, add 1 ml prewarmed PEG solution, drop-by-drop, stirring after each drop. Resuspend the pellet and let stand for 1 min.

12. Using new pipettes, add 2 ml prewarmed serum-free medium, drop-by-drop, over 2 min. Again, stir after each drop.
13. Using a 10-ml pipette, add 7 ml prewarmed medium, drop-by-drop, over 2 to 3 min.
14. Centrifuge the cells at 500*g* for 5 min at room temperature.
15. Prewarm medium with 20% FCS and CM to 37°C.
16. Discard the supernatant from Step 14. Put the centrifuge tube with the cell mixture into a 37°C water bath (place a beaker with warm water into the hood). Gently break the pellet and count the cells. Dilute the cells to a final concentration of 2.5×10^6 cells/ml in complete medium with 20% FCS and 20% CM.
17. Place 0.1 ml cell suspension into each well of 96-well flat-bottom plates.
18. Incubate overnight at 37°C in a humidified, 5% CO_2 incubator. Add 2 drops of medium with 20% FCS, 20% CM, and HAT into each well.
19. Replace the medium on days 2, 3, 4, 5, 7, 9, and 11 with complete medium with HAT.
20. On day 14, replace medium with medium with HT.
21. Cells do not require more than one change of complete medium with HT. After Step 20, and subsequently, feed cells using complete DME/F12 HYBRI-MAX medium with sodium pyruvate, amino acids, antibiotics, and 10% FCS. The cells are ready for screening when most of the wells containing growing hybridomas demonstrate 10 to 25% confluence and when those with denser populations turn yellow within 2 days after feeding.
22. Remove 0.1 ml from each well with growing cells and use it in a screening assay, such as an indirect immunofluorescence or ELISA.
23. Expand the positive wells by transferring the cells into 24-well plates and subsequently into 6-well plates.
24. Repeat screening as described in Step 22.
25. Freeze down all positive cells.
26. Select 10 to 20 best-candidate wells and clone them by limiting dilution (see below).

Comments

1. Do not stir vigorously nor pipette the cell suspension. The fused clumps are very fragile.
2. It is better to get 2 drops using a regular pipette than to use a micropipette (Step 17).
3. As a control, the parent (unfused) myeloma P653 cells should be plated in three wells at the same concentration as the myeloma cells used in the fusion. Feed following the same schedule as with the fused cells. The control myeloma cells should be dead by day 10. If these cells are not dead, either the parent myeloma cell line has reverted to a non-HAT-sensitive cell line, or the HAT used is not good.

4. Approximately 1 to 5% of the wells should contain hybridomas secreting the antibody of desired specificity.
5. Several fusion partners are available, P653 myeloma cells are probably one of the best choices.
6. Other good fusion partners are NSO/1 myeloma cells,[7] S194/5XX0 B4.1 myeloma cells,[8] and SP2/0-Ag/4 myeloma cells. SP2/0-Ag/4 is a nonsecretory myeloma that produces neither light nor heavy chains. Another advantage of this cell line is that these cells also fuse with rat and hamster B lymphocytes.
7. The use of BALB/c mice for immunization is recommended because the resulting hybridomas will be entirely of BALB/c origin and thus will form an ascites fluid in BALB/c mice.
8. Some authors[9] suggest using 20% horse serum instead of FCS. A gradual switch from horse serum to FCS might be necessary approximately 2 weeks after fusion.
9. Molecular weights of PEG from 600 to 6000 are commonly used for hybridization.
10. Some authors[6] recommend the use of a fusion solution of 42% PEG and 15% DMSO.
11. The range between 1:1 to 1:10 (myeloma cell:spleen cell) is successful.

A. *Cloning by limiting dilution*

It is quite possible that the selected hybridomas may in fact be formed by two or more clones. Similarly, they might be contaminated by a nonproducing clone. To avoid the risk of future overgrowth by these cells, cloning is necessary.

Materials and reagents

- Hybridoma cells
- Humidified, 5% CO_2 incubator
- 96-well tissue culture plate (Costar)
- 6-well tissue culture plates (Costar)
- 24-well tissue culture plates (Costar)
- DMEM medium with 10% FCS

Protocol

(*Note*: All materials and reagents must be sterile and proper aseptic techniques must be used when handling the cells.)

1. Harvest the hybridoma cells and count them.
2. Prepare two cell suspensions, 10 ml of each: 50 cells/ml and 5 cells/ml.

3. Fill one half of the wells of a 96-well plate with each dilution (0.2 ml/well).
4. Incubate for 7 to 10 days in a humidified, 5% CO_2 incubator.
5. Check the plates for cell growth. If possible, select clones from wells with a lower dilution. Look for a tight single cluster of cells.
6. Remove 0.1 ml from each well with growing cells and use it in a screening assay, such as an indirect immunofluorescence or ELISA.
7. Expand the positive wells by transferring the cells into 24-well plates, and subsequently into 6-well plates.

Comments

1. Another cloning (recloning) might be necessary. Mouse-hamster hybridomas are particularly well-known for an unstable phenotype.

B. *Growing hybridomas in dialyzing tubes*[10,11]

A well-established method for large-scale production of monoclonal antibodies is ascites production in mice. There are, however, several drawbacks to this method. First, it is rather expensive. Second, it has recently become more and more difficult to obtain permission to perform these experiments because of restrictions on the use of laboratory animals for this particular purpose. The growing of hybridomas in dialyzing tubes allows the production of monoclonal antibodies in significantly higher quantities than conventional culture in large tissue culture flasks. In addition, such supernatants contain the monoclonal antibodies in a relatively pure form, usually much purer than ascites.

Materials and reagents

- Hybridomas
- Iscove's medium (Sigma; Gibco) supplemented with 2 m*M* L-glutamine, 45 m*M* sodium pyruvate, antibiotics, 0.05% of 0.1 *M* mercaptoethanol, and 10% FCS
- FCS
- Dialyzing tube, 2.4 cm width, 12,000 to 14,000 molecular weight cutoff
- ITS Premix
- Primatone RL
- Ethanol
- Sodium bicarbonate
- EDTA-disodium
- 225-cm^2 tissue culture flasks (Costar)
- Sterile gloves

- Roller
- Sterile filtered gas mixture

Protocol

(*Note*: All materials and reagents must be sterile and proper aseptic techniques must be used when handling the cells.)

1. Prepare all media.
2. Thoroughly wash all dialyzing tubes with two washings in each of 50% ethanol, 10 mM sodium bicarbonate, 1 m*M* EDTA, and H_2O.
3. Grow the hybridomas in 225-cm^2 tissue culture flasks. One day before transfer, change the medium. Spin down the cells by centrifugation at 300*g* for 5 min at 4°C, resuspend in complete Iscove's medium, and count.
4. Resuspend 1×10^8 cells in 25 ml Iscove's medium with 2% FCS, 0.05% Primatone RL, and 0.1% ITS Premix.
5. Soak dialyzing tubes (30-cm length) in H_2O and make two knots in one end. Sterilize by boiling in H_2O for 2 hr.
6. Place sterile dialyzing tubes into a 225-cm^2 tissue culture flask and pour the cell suspension.
7. Seal the dialyzing tubes with two knots.
8. Add 60 ml Iscove's medium with 2% FCS and 0.05% Primatone RL.
9. Blow a sterile filtered gas mixture (5% CO_2 in air) into the flasks for 30 sec.
10. Place the flasks on a roller, set the revolutions to 1/5 min and incubate at 37°C in a humidified incubator.
11. Change the medium outside the dialyzing tubes and add gas every other day.
12. Harvest supernatant after 10 to 14 days of incubation.

Comments

1. The washing of dialyzing tubes is necessary to wash away all contaminants from the manufacturing process.
2. From Step 6, perform all handling under sterile conditions.
3. When two people work together, the risk of contamination is greatly reduced.
4. The speed of the roller is very important.

C. *Growing hybridomas in bioreactors*

Both laboratory practice and clinical trials reveal the growing need for large amounts of monoclonal antibodies. Antibody quantities on a scale of over 1 mg are frequently required by many laboratories. The costs of purchasing these amounts are often prohibitive. Common techniques for large-scale preparation of monoclonal antibodies are static cell culture, roller bottle cultivation, or ascites fluid. At the same time, the pressure from various animal rights groups, and even from the funding agencies, to stop production of ascites fluid is raising. On the other hand, to produce large quantities of monoclonal antibodies in normal cell cultures is laborious, time-consuming, and often difficult work. Therefore, various large-volume bioreactors have been used for large-scale production of monoclonal antibodies. As the rules of animal handling become more rigid, these modern techniques will become more and more common. Side-by-side comparisons showed that production of monoclonal antibodies in bioreactors is usually 2 to 6 times more expensive than ascites fluid. However, this is offset by the higher purity of harvested antibodies and the absence of biological contaminants.

The basic idea is simple: to significantly increase the surface area and thus allow a higher concentration of cells per unit of culture medium. The major requirements for successful long-term incubation of large quantities of cells are nutrient and gas exchange, together with pH and temperature control. After several years, bioreactors based on hollow fiber cartridges appear to offer the best solution.

Another type of bioreactor, called a modular minifermenter, has recently emerged. In this system, cells and antibodies are contained in a small disc-shaped cylinder separated from the much larger nutrient cylinder by a selective membrane. The entire module rotates around the axis of the adjacent cylinders on an apparatus similar to the one used for roller culture. At present, there is no minifermenter manufacturers in the U.S., therefore, only the hollow fiber system is described here.

D. *Growing hybridomas in hollow fiber bioreactors*

The simplistic view of hollow fiber technology is the picture of a tiny hose with uniform holes in it. The basic idea behind this technology is, in reality, quite simple: cells grow on the outside of the hollow hoses and the media can easily pass through the tiny holes. The constant flow of nutrients also enables regular removal of waste and toxic by-products. Some companies have improved upon this basic technology by flattening the fibers into sheets sandwiched between gas-permeable sheets. Using this design, much better gas delivery and pH maintenance has been achieved. The size of fiber pores used is small enough (usually a molecular weight cutoff of 10 kDa is used) so that monoclonal antibodies or other cell-secreted products are concentrated in the space outside the fiber. In addition, the pores are small even for serum; thus, fetal calf serum is added only into the extracapillary space. This experimental design has aided in reducing the need for expensive fetal calf serum. The pump generates a flow of medium and a fall in pressure along the semipermeable hollow fiber. The circulating medium is enriched with oxygen using an oxygenator. Using a silicon membrane surrounding the fibers and enclosing the extracapillary space has helped to make the diffusion route between cells and oxygen source extremely short.

In addition to large-scale production of monoclonal antibodies, hollow fiber bioreactors can be used for other functions, including cultures of endothelial and muscle cells,[12,13] production of hormones,[14] and production of other bioreactive substances.[15]

Two very similar systems exist on the current market. The first is the much bigger and more expensive Tecnomouse bioreactor offered by Integra Biosciences; the second is the similarly effective system CellMax offered by Spectrum Laboratories. The only difference (besides cost) is the fact that while CellMax can simultaneously cultivate up to four different hybridomas, Tecnomouse can simultaneously handle five. As the CellMax is significantly smaller, it easily fits into common CO_2 incubators. Tecnomouse is sold in two versions which differ in size. The larger version consists of a rather cumbersome incubator; however, the smaller version will still fill the entire CO_2 incubator. The decision to describe Tecnomouse does not suggest any preference for either of these systems.

Materials and reagents

- Tecnomouse Bioreactor (Integra Biosciences)
- CultureCassette (Integra Biosciences)
- Schott bottles with Luer lock cap (Integra Biosciences)
- 50-ml disposable syringes
- 0.2-μm sterile filters
- Iscove's medium (Sigma; Gibco) supplemented with 2 m*M* L-glutamine, 45 m*M* sodium pyruvate, antibiotics, 4.5 g/l glucose, and 1% FCS

Protocol

(*Note*: All materials and reagents must be sterile and proper aseptic techniques must be used when handling the cells.)

1. Place CultureCassette in the Tecnomouse and connect all tubing according to the manufacturer's instructions.
2. Flush the bioreactor with 2 l medium at a perfusion rate of 70 ml/hr for 24 hr.
3. Discard the medium.
4. Inoculate the CultureCassette with the hybridoma cell line precultivated to an exponentional growth phase. Prepare 5 ml cell suspension in culture medium at 5×10^7 cells/ml.
5. After cell suspension is drawn into a 10-ml syringe, connect the syringe to the left-hand port.
6. While keeping the right-hand port closed, inject the cells into the CultureCassette.
7. Replace the 2-l bottle every 7 days. First antibodies can be harvested.
8. Evaluate the antibodies using ELISA.

Comments

1. For complete information about the optimal setup and maintenance, see the manufacturer's instructions.
2. The Tecnomouse bioreactor can be used with up to five CultureCassettes hosting different hybridomas at the same time.
3. For mouse hybridomas, the manufacturer recommends using two different media:
   a. One medium for extracapillary space:
      - RPMI 1640 medium with 4.5 g/l glucose, 4 m*M* glutamine, 1% FCS, antibiotics, 1 vial OPI (Sigma)/l, and 1% Ultroser HY
   b. A second medium is for intracapillary space:
      - RPMI 1640 medium with 4.5 g/l glucose, 4 m*M* glutamine, 1% FCS, antibiotics
4. The average antibody concentration is approximately 4.5 mg/ml, with an average 75% purity.

E. *Production of ascites fluid*

Materials and reagents

- Mice
- Pristane (Sigma)
- Hybridomas
- 22-G and 18-G needles
- 5-ml syringes
- RPMI 1640 medium without FCS
- 50-ml conical centrifuge tubes
- 15-ml conical centrifuge tubes

Protocol

1. Using a 22-G needle, inject each mouse intraperitoneally with 0.5 ml Pristane 7 days prior to injection with hybridoma cells.
2. Harvest hybridoma cells, spin down by centrifugation at 350*g* for 5 min at 4°C, and count.
3. Resuspend the cells in RPMI 1640 medium without FCS to a concentration of 2.5×10^6 cells/ml.
4. Using an 18-G needle, inject each mouse intraperitoneally with 2 ml of cells.
5. Check mice periodically for formation of ascites.
6. Harvest ascites by immobilizing the mouse in one hand and inserting an 18-G needle 1 cm into the abdominal cavity. Allow the fluid to drip into 15-ml conical centrifuge tubes.

7. Mix the ascites with a wooden stick before centrifugation. Centrifuge the ascites at 1500*g* for 10 min at 4°C. Harvest supernatant and store at –20°C.

Comments

(*Note*: All materials and reagents must be sterile and proper aseptic techniques must be used when handling the cells.)

1. Use BALB/c mice (or other syngeneic strain in the case that other than usual BALB/c mice were used for original immunization). If previous attempts to produce ascites fluid failed, use more expensive athymic nude mice.
2. The total amount of cells/mouse may vary between individual hybridomas. If the mice form ascites fluid faster than 5 to 10 days after injection, decrease the number of cells in a future experiment. If no ascites fluid is formed after 3 weeks, repeat inoculation with an increased number of cells.
3. Alternatively, use mice irradiated with a sublethal dose of irradiation.
4. The ascites fluid might be under high pressure; thus, be sure that the hub of the needle is pointed into a tube before inserting into the peritoneum.
5. Repositioning or reinsertion of the needle might be necessary during harvesting of ascites fluid.
6. Wait for a full development of ascites; do not harvest the first drops of fluid.
7. Keep in mind the possibility of bioactive contaminants such as endogenous antibodies and/or cytokines.

III. Coupling of synthetic peptides to carrier proteins

Most of the synthetic peptides used for antibody production are too small to be immunogenic. In general, peptides with a length of 10 to 15 residues are used to make sera that react with the native protein. It is highly recommended to use the C-terminal sequence if the peptide is hydrophilic or the N-terminal sequence if it is hydrophobic.[16] A selected carrier protein should be a good immunogen and have a sufficient number of amino acid residues with reactive side chains. The principal carriers used most for coupling peptides include KLH (MW over 2000 kDa), bovine serum albumin (MW 67 kDa), tetanus toxoid (MW 150 kDa), ovalbumin (MW 43 kDa), and myoglobin (MW 17 kDa). Bovine serum albumin has the disadvantage that anti-carrier antibodies present in raised serum might be a problem if the serum is used in the presence of fetal calf serum.

The most commonly used reagents for peptide protein coupling are glutaraldehyde, 1-ethyl-3-(3-dimethylaminopropyl)-carbodiimide, *bis*-imido-esters, *bis*-diazotized benzidine, and *m*-maleimidobenzoyl-*N*-

hydroxysuccimide ester.[17] The choice of the coupling reagent will be based on the nature of free groups. Peptides corresponding to the amino terminus of protein should be coupled via their carboxy-terminal residue, whereas peptides corresponding to the carboxyl terminus should be coupled via their amino-terminal residue.

A. *Coupling of synthetic peptide to carrier protein using glutaraldehyde*[18]

Glutaraldehyde cross-links the carrier and peptide via their amino groups. Therefore, peptides having Lys residues at positions other than the amino terminus should not be coupled using this technique. The best KLH can be obtained from Pacific Bio-Marine Laboratories.

Materials and reagents

- Borate buffers, pH 10.0 and 8.5
- Synthetic peptide
- Keyhole limpet hemocyanin (KLH) (Calbiochem; Sigma; Pacific Bio-Marine Laboratories)
- 0.3% glutaraldehyde solution in borate buffer, pH 10.0
- 1 *M* glycine
- 15-ml glass tube
- Stir plate
- Dialyzing tube

Protocol

1. Dissolve 10 mg KLH in 2 ml borate buffer (pH 10.0), in a 15-ml glass tube. While mixing on a stir plate, add 10 mg synthetic peptide.
2. Slowly add 1 ml of 0.3% glutaraldehyde solution (freshly made) with constant mixing on a stir plate. Incubate for 2 hr at room temperature.
3. Add 0.25 ml of 1 *M* glycine to block unreacted glutaraldehyde. Incubate for 30 min at room temperature.
4. Dialyze against borate buffer (pH 8.5), overnight at 4°C. Replace with fresh borate buffer and dialyze again overnight at 4°C.

B. *Coupling of synthetic peptide to carrier protein using M-maleimidobenzoyl-N-hydroxysuccinimide ester*[18]

Materials and reagents

- *m*-Maleimidobenzoyl-*N*-hydroxysuccinimide ester (MBS; Pierce)
- Keyhole limpet hemocyanin (KLH) (Calbiochem; Sigma; Pacific Bio-Marine Laboratories)

- 0.01 *M* phosphate buffer, pH 7.0
- Dimethylformamide (Sigma)
- 0.05 M phosphate buffer, pH 6.0
- Cys-containing synthetic peptide
- PBS
- 0.1 *M* HCl
- 0.1 *M* NaOH
- Dialysis tube (10,000 molecular weight cutoff)
- 3-ml and 15-ml glass tubes
- PD-10 column (Pharmacia)
- Stir plate
- Fraction collector
- Spectrophotometer

Protocol

1. Dissolve 5 mg KLH in 0.5 ml of 0.01 *M* phosphate buffer (pH 7.0).
2. Dialyze against 0.01 *M* phosphate buffer (pH 7.0), overnight at 4°C. Put the dialyzed solution into a 3-ml glas tube.
3. Add 70 μl of 15 mg/ml MBS in dimethylformamide (prepared fresh) to the dialyzed solution and gently mix on a stir plate for 30 min at room temperature.
4. Prepare a PD-10 column by washing with 50 ml of 0.05 *M* phosphate buffer (pH 6.0). Load the mixture from Step 3 and elute with 0.05 *M* phosphate buffer (pH 6.0). Collect 0.5-ml fractions and check the A_{280} of these fractions. The first peak represents maleimide-activated KLH; the second peak represents free MBS.
5. Pool the maleimide-activated KLH fractions in a 15-ml glass tube.
6. Dissolve 5 mg synthetic peptide in 1 ml PBS.
7. Mix the pooled fraction with the peptide solution. Adjust pH to 7.3 and incubate for 3 hr at room temperature with constant mixing.
8. Dialyze against water overnight at 4°C. Replace with fresh water and dialyze overnight again at 4°C.

Comments

1. If the peptide is not soluble in PBS, try 6 *M* guanidine-HCl/0.01 *M* phosphate buffer (pH 7.0).

C. Coupling of synthetic peptide to carrier protein using 1-ethyl-3-(3-dimethylaminopropyl)carbodiimide

1-Ethyl-3-(3-dimethylaminopropyl)carbodiimide cross-links the free amino acid group of a carrier with a C-terminal carboxyl group of the peptide. Do not use peptides with internal Asp, Glu, or Lys residues.

Materials and reagents

- 1-Ethyl-3-(3-dimethylaminopropyl)carbodiimide-HCl (EDCI; Sigma)
- 5-ml glass tube
- Synthetic peptide
- Keyhole limpet hemocyanin (KLH((Calbiochem; Sigma; Pacific Bio-Marine Laboratories)
- Stir plate
- Dialysis tube (10,000 molecular weight cutoff)

Protocol

1. Dissolve 10 mg peptide in 1 ml H_2O in a 5-ml glass tube.
2. Add 40 mg EDCI to this solution with constant gentle stirring. Adjust pH to 4.5 and incubate for 10 min at room temperature.
3. Add 0.5 ml KLH (5 mg/ml in water) to this solution. Incubate for 2 hr at room temperature.
4. Dialyze against water overnight at 4°C. Replace with fresh water and dialyze again overnight at 4°C.

D. *Coupling of synthetic peptide to carrier protein using* bis-*diazotized benzidine*[18]

Bis-diazotized benzidine cross-links Tyr residues in the carrier protein to Tyr residues in peptides.

Materials and reagents

- Benzidine-HCl (Sigma)
- 0.2 *M* HCl
- $NaNO_2$
- Borate buffer, pH 9.0
- 15-ml test tube
- Beaker
- Keyhole limpet hemocyanin (KLH) (Calbiochem; Sigma; Pacific Bio-Marine Laboratories)
- Synthetic peptide
- Dialyzing tube
- Stir plate
- Ice

Protocol

1. Dissolve 5 mg benzidine in 1 ml of 0.2 *M* HCl. Add 3.5 mg $NaNO_2$ and incubate 1 hr with constant stirring at 4°C in the dark.

2. Dissolve 5 mg KLH in 10 ml borate buffer (pH 9.0), in a beaker. Add 2 mg synthetic peptide and cool on ice.
3. Add dropwise a *bis*-diazotized benzidine solution from Step 1 to the solution from Step 2. Adjust pH to 9.0 and incubate with constant stirring for 2 hr at 4°C.
4. Dialyze against water overnight at 4°C. Replace with fresh water and dialyze overnight again at 4°C.

Comments

1. Benzidine and *bis*-diazotized benzidine are carcinogens.

IV. Purification of immunoglobulins

Several excellent and detailed reviews and monographs describing isolation and characterization of immunoglobulins have been published.[19-21] Extinction coefficients and molecular size of immunoglobulins and their fragments are shown in Table 9.1.

Table 9.1 Extinction Coefficients and Molecular Size of Immunoglobulins and Their Fragments

		Molecular Weight (kDa)		
	A_{280}	Nonreduced	Reduced	
Molecule	(1 mg/ml)		Heavy Chain	Light Chain
IgG	1.43	160	55	25
IgM	1.18	900	78	25
Fab	1.53	50	25	25
$F(ab)_2$	1.48	100–110	25	25
$F(ab)_2$:μ	1.38	135	44	25
F(ab):μ	1.38	65	44	25

A. Precipitation by ammonium sulfate

Materials and reagents

- Saturated $(NH_4)_2SO_4$ (SAS)
- Glass beaker
- Magnetic stirrer
- Serum or ascites fluid
- Hotplate
- Dialysis tube
- Glass pipette
- Sodium azide
- PBS
- Spectrophotometer

Protocol

1. To make SAS, dissolve approximately 900 g ammonium sulfate in 1000 ml boiling H_2O. Let the solution cool to room temperature. Crystals of $(NH_4)_2SO_4$ will form and should always be present.
2. Clarify serum or ascites fluid by centrifugation at 10,000*g* for 30 min at 4°C. Decant and save the supernatant; discard membranous material and cell debris remaining in the pellet.
3. Place supernatant into a beaker and begin stirring. Add SAS slowly until precipitate starts to form. Then slowly bring up to 50% (vol/vol) SAS. Allow precipitate to form for an additional 2 to 4 hr at 4°C or overnight.
4. Centrifuge at 10,000*g* for 60 min at 4°C and save precipitate. Save the supernatant to check for residual antibody activity.
5. Dissolve precipitate in a minimum (usually less than 50% of the original) volume of PBS.
6. Measure the concentration of IgG at OD_{280}.
7. Dialyze against PBS (or desired buffer) overnight at 4°C. Add sodium azide to 10 m*M* and store at 4°C or use for further purification.

Comments

1. Removal of lipids by a passage of ascites fluid over a funnel with glass wool might be necessary before performing Step 2.

B. *Caprylic acid-ammonium sulfate isolation of IgG from ascites fluid*

Materials and reagents

- Ascites fluid
- Caprylic acid (Sigma)
- Fumehood
- Centrifuge tubes
- Saturated $(NH_4)_2SO_4$ (SAS)
- PBS
- Dialysis tube
- Sodium azide
- Acetic acid
- Stirring plate
- pH meter

Protocol

1. Adjust the pH of the ascites fluid to 4.95 using 3 *M* acetic acid. The correct pH is extremely important.

2. While stirring at room temperature under the fumehood, slowly add caprylic acid to a final concentration of 5% (1:20).
3. Stir for 30 min at room temperature.
4. Centrifuge at 10,000*g* for 30 min at 20°C.
5. The supernatant contains the antibody; thus, save supernatant and discard precipitate.
6. Measure the volume of the supernatant.
7. Slowly add an equal volume of SAS while stirring at room temperature.
8. Stir for 2 hr at 4°C.
9. Centrifuge as in Step 4.
10. Decant supernatant and discard; save precipitate.
11. Blot tube well to remove as much ammonium sulfate as possible.
12. Redissolve precipitate in a minimum volume of PBS (usually less than 50% volume of original ascites).
13. Dialyze overnight against PBS (or other desired buffer) at 4°C to remove residual ammonium sulfate.
14. Centrifuge again as in Step 4 to remove undissolved precipitate.
15. Either add sodium azide to 10 m*M* and store the antibody at 4°C or freeze at –80°C.

Comments

1. Use polycarbonate, polysulfone, nylon, or glass centrifuge tubes because the caprylic acid will dissolve polyethylene, polystyrene, and polypropylene plastic tubes.

C. *Purification of antibodies by precipitation with polyethylene glycol*[22,23]

Different monoclonal antibodies precipitate out at different concentrations of polyethylene glycol (PEG). In general, the higher the concentration of the PEG used, the higher the resulting contamination of the sample. Some IgG and most IgM antibodies precipitate out below 5% PEG.

Materials and reagents

- Polyethylene glycol 6000 (PEG)
- Ascites fluid
- Veronal buffered saline (VBS)
- Centrifuge tubes
- Eppendorf microtubes
- Electrophoresis equipment

Protocol

1. Clarify ascites fluid by centrifugation at 10,000*g* for 30 min at 4°C. Decant and save the supernatant; discard membranous material and cell debris remaining in the pellet.

2. Prepare stock solutions (w/v) of 0%, 4%, 8%, 12%, 16%, 20%, 24%, 28%, 32%, and 50% PEG in VBS. Store them at 4°C.
3. To determine the optimal concentration of PEG for a particular antibody, perform a pilot test. Place 20 µl cold clarified ascites fluid into Eppendorf microtubes and add 20 µl of different concentrations of PEG.
4. Mix the tubes and incubate them for 30 min on ice. Spin the tubes at 2000*g* for 20 min at 4°C.
5. Test the supernatant for the presence of the monoclonal antibody band. The concentration of PEG that removed most of the antibody band is the optimal concentration.
6. Perform the same experiment on a large scale using only the optimal concentration of PEG.

Comments

1. Step 6 can be repeated to achieve higher purity. Unlike ammonium sulfate precipitation, multiple precipitations in PEG and redissolving do not affect their functional characteristics.

D. Purification of antibodies from culture supernatants by precipitation with polyethylene glycol[22]

Materials and reagents

- Polyethylene glycol 6000 (PEG)
- Tissue culture supernatant
- Veronal buffered saline (VBS)
- Centrifugation tubes
- Electrophoresis equipment
- 0.3 *M* phosphate buffer, pH 6.8

Protocol

1. Clarify culture supernatant by centrifugation at 10,000*g* for 30 min at 4°C. Decant and save the supernatant; discard membranous material and cell debris remaining in the pellet.
2. Add solid PEG at 12.5% (w/v) concentration to cold clarified culture supernatant.
3. Stir until all the PEG is dissolved.
4. Incubate overnight at 4°C.
5. Collect the precipitate by centrifugation at 2000*g* for 20 min at 4°C.
6. Dissolve the precipitate in 2% of the original volume VBS. Incubate for 2 hr at 4°C.
7. Centrifuge at 2000*g* for 20 min at 4°C.

8. Collect the supernatant. Dissolve the pellet with 1% original volume of culture supernatant with 0.3 *M* phosphate buffer (pH 6.8).
9. Centrifuge at 2000*g* for 20 min at 4°C.
10. Test for the presence of antibodies by electrophoresis.
11. Isolate the monoclonal antibodies by performing Steps 3 to 6 from the previous method.

Comments

1. Serum-free tissue culture supernatants cannot be purified using this method due to the low concentration of proteins, which does not allow effective PEG precipitation.

E. *Affinity chromatography using Protein A-Sepharose*[19,24]

Materials and reagents

- Tissue culture supernatant or ascites fluid
- 1 *M* NaOH
- Protein A-Sepharose CL-4B (Pharmacia)
- 0.1 *M* citric acid
- 3 *M* potassium thiocyanate
- 1.5 × 10-cm glass column
- Fraction collector
- Dialysis tubing
- PBS, pH 8.0
- Spectrophotometer

Protocol

1. Clarify culture supernatant or ascites fluid by centrifugation at 10,000*g* for 30 min at 4°C. Decant and save the supernatant; discard membranous material and cell debris remaining in the pellet.
2. Dilute ascites fluid 10× with PBS (pH 8.0), or adjust tissue culture supernatant to pH 8.0 by dialysis against PBS (pH 8.0), overnight at 4°C.
3. Prepare Protein A-Sepharose column and attach a fraction collector.
4. Equilibrate column with PBS (pH 8.0), at 4°C.
5. Load the column with supernatant/ascites fluid.
6. Wash the column with several volumes of PBS (pH 8.0).
7. Check OD_{280} of the eluate. Keep washing until the OD_{280} is at the baseline.
8. Elute IgG with 0.1 M citric acid at pH optimal for desired isotype. For mouse IgG, use pH 6.5; for IgG_{2a}, use pH 4.5; and for IgG_{2b} and IgG_3, use pH 3.0.
9. Pool fractions containing immunoglobulins (check OD_{280}). Put the eluates into dialysis tubing and dialyze against PBS (pH 7.3), with 0.02% NaN_3 overnight at 4°C.

10. Clean the column with 1 volume of filtered 3 *M* potassium thiocyanate. Reequilibrate the column in PBS using several volumes of PBS (pH 7.3). Store at 4°C.

Comments

1. Most mouse and human IgG antibodies bind to Protein A.
2. The binding capacity of a Protein A-Sepharose column is approximately 5 mg mouse IgG and 8 mg human IgG per 1 ml of Protein A-Sepharose.

F. *Purification of IgM*[19,20]

Materials and reagents

- IgM
- Borate buffer
- Dialysis tube
- Size-exclusion (SE) column
- SDS-PAGE electrophoresis
- Fraction collector

Protocol

1. Dialyze antibody against H_2O at 4°C for 24 hr.
2. Centrifuge dialyzed antibody at 20,000*g* at 4°C for 60 min. Discard supernatant and dissolve pellet in 5 ml borate buffer.
3. Prepare an SE column and equilibrate with borate buffer. Add antibody and elute with borate buffer. Collect 100 fractions. IgM will be in the first protein peak.
4. Measure IgM concentration at OD_{280}.
5. Check the purity of the IgM on a 10% SDS-PAGE gel under reducing conditions.
6. Store in borate buffer at 4°C or at –70°C.

Comments

1. Most IgM antibodies are not soluble in water.

G. *Ammonium sulfate precipitation of IgM*[19,20]

Materials and reagents

- Saturated $(NH_4)_2SO_4$ (SAS)
- Glass beaker
- Magnetic stirrer

- Serum or ascites fluid
- Spectrophotometer
- Size-exclusion (SE) column
- SDS-PAGE electrophoresis
- Borate buffer
- Fraction collector

Protocol

1. Clarify serum or ascites fluid by centrifugation at 10,000*g* for 30 min at 4°C. Decant and save the supernatant; discard membranous material and cell debris remaining in the pellet.
2. Put supernatant into a beaker and begin stirring. Add SAS slowly to 45% (v/v) antibody. Allow precipitate to form for an additional 2 to 4 hr or overnight at 4°C .
3. Centrifuge at 10,000*g* for 60 min at 4°C and save precipitate. Save the supernatant to check for residual antibody activity.
4. Dissolve precipitate in a minimum (usually less than 50% of the original volume) volume of borate buffer.
5. Prepare an SE column and equlibrate with borate buffer. Add antibody and elute with borate buffer. Collect 100 fractions. IgM will be in the first protein peak.
6. Measure IgM concentration at OD_{280}.
7. Check the purity of the IgM on a 10% SDS-PAGE gel under reducing conditions.
8. Store in borate buffer at 4°C or at –70°C.

Comments

1. Use for IgM antibodies that do not precipitate in water.

H. Purification of anti-hapten antibodies by affinity chromatography

This procedure describes purification of anti-Arsonate (Ars) antibodies.[25] One can either activate agarose with CNBr[26] or use commercially available CNBr-activated agarose.

Materials and reagents

- Stirring plate
- CNBr-activated agarose (Pharmacia)
- $NaHCO_3$ buffer
- Glass beaker
- Parafilm™
- Sintered glass funnel
- PBS
- H_2O

- Acetic acid
- Column
- Sodium azide (NaN_3)
- Anti-serum
- Spectrophotometer

Protocol

1. Add 1 ml Ars (40 m*M* solution in 0.1 *M* $NaHCO_3$, pH 9.0 buffer) to 10 ml CNBr-activated agarose in glass beaker. Cover the beaker with Parafilm and stir the mixture slowly for 24 hr at 4°C.
2. Transfer the CNBr-activated agarose to a sintered glass funnel and wash with 1 l ice-cold H_2O, followed by 1 l ice-cold 0.1 *M* $NaHCO_3$, pH 9.0 buffer. Resuspend CNBr-activated agarose in PBS.
3. Put CNBr-activated agarose into a suitable column. Slowly add the anti-serum to the column and collect the eluate. 10 ml of CNBr-activated agarose will bind approximately 200 mg of specific antibody.
4. Wash the column with PBS until the eluate has an OD_{280} of less than 0.01.
5. Combine all eluted fractions, concentrate, and dialyze against PBS overnight at 4°C. Determine the amount of antibody by measuring the absorbance at 280 nm.

Comments

1. The column can be reused. It is necessary to remove all antibodies from the column by washing with 2 volumes of 0.1 *M* acetic acid before reuse. Equilibrate the column with 2 l of PBS and store at 4°C with 0.02% sodium azide.

I. Fragmentation of immunoglobulin into F(ab) fragments using papain

Papain specifically digests IgG into F(ab) fragments. This technique can be used for every subclass of IgG molecule.

Materials and reagents

- 2 mg/ml purified antibody in PBS
- Papain (2X crystallized suspension; Sigma Cat. No. P3125)
- Digestion buffer
- PBS
- 0.3 *M* iodoacetamide (prepare fresh from crystalline material) in PBS
- Eppendorf microcentrifuge tubes

- Water bath
- SDS-PAGE electrophoresis
- Dialysis tube
- Glass Pasteur pipette
- Burner
- Spectrophotometer
- Vortex

Protocol

1. Determine protein concentration of purified antibody (OD at 280 nm).
2. Pipette 100 µl of 2 mg/ml purified IgG in PBS into each of 13 numbered microcentrifuge tubes.
3. Prepare two papain solutions in 5 ml digestion buffer: one at 0.02 mg/ml papain and the other at 0.04 mg/ml papain.
4. Add 100 µl of 0.02 mg/ml papain to six of the IgG tubes. Add 100 µl of 0.04 mg/ml papain to a second group of six IgG tubes. Finally, add 100 µl of digestion buffer without papain to one of the IgG tubes.
5. Prepare a digestion time curve by incubating tubes in a 37°C water bath and removing them at different times in groups of two (one tube each of enzyme:antibody ratio at 1:20 and 1:100). Remove the first group after 1 hr and subsequent groups at 2, 4, 5, 6, and 24 hr. Remove the control tube with the 24-hr set. As each group is removed from the water bath, terminate the reaction by adding 20 µl of 0.3 *M* iodoacetamide in PBS and then vortexing.
6. Puncture the lid of another set of microcentrifuge tubes using a heated glass Pasteur pipette (wide end heated) to completely remove the center part of the lid. Pipette contents of reaction tubes into similarly labeled dialysis tubes. Open the lid, place a single layer of dialysis tubing over the top of the tube, and then close the lid to hold dialysis tubing in place.
7. Turn tube upside down and shake reaction mixture onto the membrane surface. Tape each tube, dialysis surface down, to the side of a beaker filled with PBS and dialyze 4 hr at 4°C with stirring.
8. Analyze digestion products by running 12.5% nonreducing SDS-PAGE electrophoresis.

J. Fragmentation of immunoglobulin into F(ab) fragments using preactivated papain[19]

This technique is a gentler method than the one described above. Thus, it is not necessary to perform a pilot experiment.

Materials and reagents

- 10 mg IgG in 5 ml PBS
- Acetate/EDTA buffer
- 2 mg/ml papain acetate/EDTA buffer
- 0.05 *M* cysteine (free base, Sigma)
- Iodoacetamine crystals
- PD-10 column (Pharmacia)
- Dialysis tube
- Water bath
- PBS, pH 8.0
- Protein A-Sepharose column
- Size-exclusion (SE) column
- SDS-PAGE electrophoresis
- PBS containing 0.02% NaN_3
- Spectrophotometer
- Fraction collector
- Amicon concentrator

Protocol

1. Dialyze IgG in acetate/EDTA buffer at 4°C overnight.
2. Determine the concentration of antibody at OD_{280}.
3. Incubate 2 mg/ml papain and 0.05 *M* cysteine for 30 min in a 37°C water bath.
4. Equilibrate a PD-10 column with 20 ml acetate/EDTA buffer.
5. Apply papain/cystein mixture to the PD-10 column. Elute with acetate/EDTA buffer and collect ten 1-ml fractions.
6. Check the fractions at OD_{280} and pool three (3) fractions containing papain. Calculate the preactivated papain concentration:

$$A_{280}/2.5 = \text{mg preactivated papain}$$

7. Add 0.5 mg preactivated papain to purified IgG in acetate/EDTA buffer. Shake and incubate 10 hr in a 37°C water bath.
8. Add crystalline iodoacetamine to a final concentration of 0.03 *M*.
9. Dialyze against PBS (pH 8.0), at 4°C overnight.
10. Calibrate a Protein A-Sepharose column with PBS (pH 8.0). Add papain/IgG mixture. Collect unbound 2-ml fractions. Pool fractions forming the first peak and concentrate to a volume less than 5 ml.
11. Load the sample onto an SE column. Collect 100 fractions and check the molecular weight of fractions using SDS-PAGE electrophoresis.
12. Store in PBS containing 0.02% NaN_3 at –70°C.

K. *Fragmentation of immunoglobulin into F(ab')$_2$ fragments using pepsin*

Pepsin is used for a fragmentation of IgG into F(ab')$_2$ fragments. The optimal pH for pepsin is around 2; because since it would be damaging for the antibodies, a pH of 4.1 is used. Do not use this method for F(ab')$_2$ fragmentation of IgG$_{2b}$, as Fab/c fragments will be produced.

Materials and reagents

- Purified antibody
- 0.1 *M* sodium acetate buffer, pH 4.1
- Dialyzing tubes
- Pepsin (Sigma)
- 1 *M* Trizma base
- 0.5 *M* NaCl
- 0.05 *M* phosphate buffer, pH 7.3
- Amicon concentrator
- Eppendorf microcentrifuge tubes
- Water bath
- Electrophoresis
- S-200 column (Pharmacia)
- Fraction collector
- Spectrophotometer

Protocol

1. Dialyze purified antibody overnight against 0.1 *M* sodium acetate buffer (pH 4.1), at 4°C.
2. Determine protein concentration of purified antibody (OD at 280 nm).
3. Dilute antibody to 5 mg/ml in 0.1 *M* sodium acetate buffer. Put 0.2 ml of the diluted antibody into Eppendorf microcentrifuge tubes.
4. Prepare fresh pepsin at an exact concentration of 1 mg/ml in 0.1 *M* sodium acetate buffer (pH 4.1).
5. Use pepsin-to-antibody percentages of:
   a. 0.1% (0.1 μl pepsin to 100 μg/ml of antibody)
   b. 0.2% (0.2 μl pepsin to 100 μg/ml of antibody)
   c. 1.0% (1.0 μl pepsin to 100 μg/ml of antibody)
   d. 2.0% (2.0 μl pepsin to 100 μg/ml of antibody)
   e. 5.0% (5.0 μl pepsin to 100 μg/ml of antibody)
6. Digest for 7 hr at 37°C.
7. Add an equal volume of 1 *M* Trizma base to each tube to stop digestion.
8. Run an SDS electrophoresis to determine the percentage of F(ab')$_2$ fragments.
9. Use the optimal dose of pepsin on a large-scale experiment.

10. Reconcentrate to 10 mg/ml using an Amicon concentrator.
11. Equilibrate an S-200 column of around 1 m length with 0.05 *M* phosphate buffer (pH 7.3), and 0.5 *M* NaCl.
12. Run the sample (up to 15 ml) through the column.
13. Collect, monitor (OD at 280 nm), and plot fractions. The $F(ab')_2$ will elute following the undigested antibody.

Comments

1. The pH of 0.1 *M* sodium acetate buffer is very critical.
2. The optimal concentration of pepsin depends on several factors such as the antibody, activity of the pepsin, etc. Therefore, it is necessary to perform a pilot experiment prior to a large-scale digestion.

L. *Double immunodiffusion assay*[27]

The double immunodiffusion assay is a simple method for detecting the presence of antigen-specific antibodies. Solutions of antigen and antibody are placed in adjacent wells and allowed to diffuse into the gel. In case of an antigen-antibody reaction, an immunoprecipitation line will form between the wells containing antigen and antigen-specific antibody.

Materials and reagents

- PBS
- Anti-sera
- Antigen
- Staining solution
- Destaining solution
- Agarose
- Microscope slides
- Ouchterlony template
- Aspirator
- Coplin jar
- Filter paper
- 37°C incubator

Protocol

1. Melt 1% agarose and apply no more than 3.3 ml agarose to the slide (keep slides on a level surface).
2. Allow agarose to harden, but do not allow it to dry. If the slide is to be out awhile, place it in a wet box.
3. Place slide on an Ouchterlony template and punch holes in the agarose.
4. Carefully remove the slide from the template. Remove the agarose plugs with the aspirator.

5. Make serial dilutions of the antigen in PBS.
6. Place approximately 12 μl antigen in each of the outer wells. The volume will vary according to how much agarose was applied to the slide. Fill each well to the top.
7. In the center well, add approximately 25 μl of antibody (also filling it to the top).
8. Place the slides in the wet box and incubate it at 4°C for 2 days. Initial results may be seen in just a few hours; but to develop completely, the slides should be allowed to develop for 2 days.
9. After the 48-hr incubation, place slides in a Coplin jar filled with PBS for 2 days.
10. Remove slides from PBS and place filter paper over the agarose, wrapping the edges of the filter paper around the slide. Place in 37°C incubator and bake for approximately 2 hr to dry the agarose.
11. Stain slides in staining solution for 10 min.
12. Destain for 4 min in destaining solution. Remove slides and place in fresh destaining solution for another 4 min.

References

1. Bennet, B., Check, I.J., Olsen, M.R., and Hunter, R.L., A comparison of commercially available adjuvants for use in research, *J. Immunol. Methods*, 153, 31, 1992.
2. Kohler, G. and Milstein, C., Continuous cultures of fused cells secreting antibody of predefined specificity, *Nature*, 256, 495, 1975.
3. Springer, T.A., Ed., in *Hybridoma Technology in the Biosciences and Medicine*, Plenum Press, New York, 1985.
4. Goding, J.W., *Monoclonal Antibodies: Principles and Practise*, Academic Press, San Diego, 1986.
5. Oi, V.T. and Herzenberg, L.A., Immunoglobulin-producing hybrid cell lines, in *Selected Methods in Cellular Immunology*, Mishell, B.B. and Shiigi, S.M., Eds., W.H. Freeman, New York, 1980, 351.
6. Zola, H., *Monoclonal Antibodies: A Manual of Techniques*, CRC Press, Boca Raton, FL, 1985.
7. Galfre, G. and Milstein, C., Preparation of monoclonal antibodies: Strategies and procedures, *Meth. Enzymol.*, 73, 3, 1981.
8. Trowbridge, I.S., Interspecies spleen myeloma hybrid producing monoclonal antibodies against mouse lymphocyte surface glycoprotein T200, *J. Exp. Med.*, 148, 313, 1978.
9. Eshhar, Z., Monoclonal antibody strategy and techniques, in *Hybridoma Technology in the Biosciences and Medicine*, Springer, T.A., Ed., Plenum Press, New York, 1985, 3.
10. Sjogren-Jansson, E. and Jeansson, S., Growing hybridomas in dialysis tubing: optimalization of the technique, in *Laboratory Methods in Immunology*, Vol. I, Zola, H., Ed., CRC Press, Boca Raton, FL, 1990, 41.
11. Sjogren-Jansson, E. and Jeansson, S., Large-scale production of monoclonal antibodies in dialysis tubing, *J. Immunol. Methods*, 84, 359, 1985.

12. Redmond, E.M., Cahill, P.A., and Sitzmann, J.V., Perfused transcapillary smooth muscle and endothelial cell co-culture — a novel *in vitro* model, *In Vitro Dev. Biol.*, 31, 601, 1995.
13. Ott, M.J., Olson, J.L., and Ballermann, B.J., Chronic *in vitro* flow promotes ultrastructural differentiation of endothelial cells, *Endothelium*, 3, 21, 1995.
14. Knazek, R. A., Kohler, P. P., and Gullino, P. M., Hormone production by cells grown *in vitro* on artificial capillaries, *Exp. Cell Res.*, 84, 251, 1974.
15. Packard, B. C. and Komoriya, A., A 36-kilodalton tumor-derived factor with myeloid immunomodulatory activity, *J. Biol. Chem.*, 268, 6356, 1993.
16. Maloy, W.L. and Coligan, J.E. Selection of immunogenic peptides for antisera production, in *Current Protocols in Immunology*, Coligan, J.E., Kruisbeek, A.M., Margulies, D.H., Shevach, E.M., and Strober, W., Eds., Greene Publishing and Wiley InterScience, New York, 1994, 9.3.1.
17. Van Regenmortel, M.H.V., Briand, J.P., Muller, S. and Plaue, S., Synthetic polypeptides as antigens, in *Laboratory Techniques in Biochemistry and Molecular Biology*, Vol. 19, Burdon, R.H. and von Knippenberg, P.H., Eds., Elsevier, Amsterdam, 1988, 361.
18. Maloy, W.L., Coligan, J.E. and Paterson, Y., Production of antipeptide antisera, in *Current Protocols in Immunology*, Coligan, J.E., Kruisbeek, A M., Margulies, D.H., Shevach, E.M., and Strober, W., Eds., Greene Publishing and Wiley InterScience, New York, 1991, 9.4.1.
19. Andrew, S.M. and Titus, J.A., Purification of antibodies and preparation of antibody fragments, in *Current Protocols in Immunology*, Colignan, J.E., Kruisbeek, A.M., Margulies, D.H., Shevach, E.M., and Strober, W., Eds., Greene Publishing and Wiley InterScience, New York, 1992, 2.7.1.
20. Hardy, R.R., Purification and characterization of monoclonal antibodies, in *Handbook of Experimental Immunology, Vol. 1, Immunochemistry*, Weir, D.M., Ed., Blackwell Scientific, Oxford, 1986, 13.1.
21. Kabat, E.A., *Structural Concepts in Immunology and Immunochemistry*, 2nd ed., Holt, Reinhart & Winston, New York, 1976.
22. Neoh, S. and Zola, H., Purification of mouse monoclonal antibodies from ascitic fluid and culture supernatants by precipitation with polyethylene glycol 6000, in *Laboratory Methods in Immunology*, Zola, H., Ed., CRC Press, Boca Raton, FL, 1990, 73.
23. Neoh, S.H., Gordon, C., Potter, A., and Zola, G., The purification of mouse monoclonal antibodies from ascitic fluid, *J. Immunol. Meth.*, 91, 231, 1986.
24. Ey, P.L., Prouse, S.J., and Jenkin, C.R., Isolation of pure IgG_1, IgG_{2a}, and IgG_{2b} immunoglobulins from mouse serum using protein A-Sepharose, *Immunochemistry*, 15, 429, 1978.
25. Wofsy, L. and Burr, B., The use of affinity chromatography for the specific purification of antibodies and antigens, *J. Immunol.*, 103, 380, 1969.
26. Hood, A.H., Wofsy, L., Kimura, J., and Henry, C., Purification of immunoglobulins and their fragments, in *Selected Methods in Cellular Immunology*, Mishell, B.B. and Shiigi, S.M., Eds., W.H. Freeman, San Francisco, 1980, 278.
27. Ouchterlony, O. and Nilsson, L.A., Immunodiffusion and immunoelectrophoresis, in *Handbook of Experimental Immunology, Vol. 1., Immunochemistry*, Weir, D.M., Herzenberg, L.A., and Blackwell, C., Eds., Blackwell, Oxford, 1986, 32.1.

chapter ten

ELISA

Contents

Enzyme-linked immunosorbent assay (ELISA)[1] is a technique for assaying the presence of antibodies in various fluids. Using any of numerous modifications, this method allows one to qualitatively or quantitatively evaluate a particular antibody activity, to measure an antigen using a defined antibody preparation, or to detect cell-surface antigens. ELISA is one of the most versatile and widely used techniques, and its sensitivity is between 100 pg/ml and 1 ng/ml.

As a general rule, the incubation times used in individual steps might be either overnight at 4°C, or 2 hr at either room temperature or 37°C. The term *incubate* is used instead of repeating "overnight at 4°C or 2 hr at either room temperature or 37°C" in every step.

It is very difficult to find two laboratories performing this assay exactly the same way. Readers should try to use the following information as a basis for development of their own modification. One of the more important modifications is the use of 0.25% gelatin or 5% instant milk instead of bovine serum albumin.

Various substrates used for visualization of an ELISA assays are shown in Table 10.1.

Table 10.1 Various Substrates Used for Visualization of an ELISA

Enzyme	Substrate	OD (nm)
Alkaline phosphatase[a]	*p*-Nitrophenyl phosphate	405
	4-Methylumbelliferyl phosphate	365/450
Horseradish peroxidase	*o*-Phenylendiamine	492
	2,2′-Azino-*bis*-(3-ethylbenzthiazoline Sulfonic acid	414
	o-Dianisidine	530
	5-Aminosalicylic acid	474
	3,3′,5,5′-Tetramethylbenzidine	450
β-D-galactosidase	*o*-Nitrophenyl-β-D-galactopyranoside	420
	Chlorophenolic red-β-D-Galactopyranoside	574
	Resorufin-β-D-Galactopyranoside	570
Urease	Bromcresol purple	588
Acetylcholine esterase	Ellman's reagent	412

[a]The fluorogenic system using 4-methylumbelliferyl phosphate is up to 100 times faster than using *p*-nitrophenyl phosphate.

Note: Readers seeking more information about various enzyme-substrate combinations should see reference 2.

I. Indirect ELISA

This technique is used primarily for screening antibodies such as in testing of hybridoma culture supernatants. It does not require the use of preexisting specific antibodies. The wells are coated with the antigen, followed by incubation with supernatants. Unbound antibodies are washed out and an Ig-specific antibody conjugated to an enzyme is used for visualization.

Materials and reagents

- ELISA reader
- Antigen
- Test samples
- Enzyme-conjugated antibody
- 96-well U- or flat-bottom microtiter plates (Immulon; Dynatech)
- Substrate
- PBS containing 0.05% Tween 20 (PBS-Tween)
- PBS containing 0.05% Tween 20, 1% BSA, and 0.02% NaN_3 (PBS-BSA-Tween)
- Multichannel pipette

- Carbonate-bicarbonate buffer, pH 9.6
- Plastic squirt bottle
- Paper towels

Protocol

1. Dilute the antigen in carbonate-bicarbonate buffer at a concentration of 5 μg/ml. Using a multichannel pipette, dispense 100 μl of antigen solution into each well on each plate. This coats the plates with antigen.
2. Cover the plates with a cover or wrap them in plastic wrap and incubate them.
3. Rinse the plates 5× over a sink by filling all wells with PBS-Tween from a plastic squirt bottle. Flick the PBS-Tween into the sink after each rinse.
4. Block residual binding capacity of wells by filling all wells with PBS-BSA-Tween and incubating for 30 min at room temperature.
5. Rinse the plates 5× over a sink by filling all wells with PBS-Tween from a plastic squirt bottle. Flick the PBS-Tween into the sink after each rinse. After the last wash, remove residual PBS-Tween by laying the plates face down on paper towels for several seconds.
6. Add 100 μl of test samples diluted in PBS-BSA-Tween to each well. Cover the plates and incubate.
7. Rinse the plates 5× over a sink by filling all wells with PBS-Tween from a plastic squirt bottle. Flick the PBS-Tween into the sink after each rinse. After the last wash, remove residual PBS-Tween by laying the plates face down on paper towels for several seconds.
8. Add 100 μl of enzyme-conjugated antibody diluted in PBS-BSA-Tween to each well. Cover the plates and incubate.
9. Rinse the plates 3× over a sink by filling all wells with PBS-Tween from a plastic squirt bottle. Flick the PBS-Tween into the sink after each rinse. After the last wash, remove residual PBS-Tween by laying the plates face down on paper towels for several seconds.
10. Add 100 μl of substrate solution to each well, cover the plates, and incubate them for 1 hr at room temperature in the dark. Check the color development occasionally. Read the reaction on an ELISA reader using the appropriate filter.

Comments

1. The optimal concentration of enzyme-conjugated antibody should be determined by a pilot experiment utilizing criss-cross serial dilution analysis.
2. Covered antigen-coated plates can be stored at 4°C for several months. Do not let them dry out.

3. The optimal incubation time in Step 10 depends on the type of enzyme-substrate combination and on the concentration of antibody in tested samples. Stop the reaction (either by reading or by adding a stopping reagent) when positive wells reach the desired intensity.

II. Antibody-sandwich ELISA for detection of soluble antigens

The wells are coated with a specific antibody followed by incubation with antigen-containing solutions. Unbound material is washed out and different enzyme-conjugated antigen-specific antibodies are used for visualization.

Materials and reagents

- ELISA reader
- Specific antibody
- Tested solution
- Enzyme-conjugated antibody
- 96-well U- or flat-bottom microtiter plates (Immulon; Dynatech)
- Substrate
- PBS containing 0.05% Tween 20 (PBS-Tween)
- PBS containing 0.05% Tween 20, 1% BSA, and 0.02% NaN_3 (PBS-BSA-Tween)
- Multichannel pipette
- Carbonate-bicarbonate buffer, pH 9.6
- Plastic squirt bottle
- Paper towels

Protocol

1. Dilute the specific antibody in carbonate-bicarbonate buffer at a concentration of 5 μg/ml. Using a multichannel pipette, dispense 100 μl of antibody solution into each well on each plate. This coats the plates with the specific antibody.
2. Cover the plates with a cover or wrap them in plastic wrap and incubate them.
3. Rinse the plates 5× over a sink by filling all wells with PBS-Tween from a plastic squirt bottle. Flick the PBS-Tween into the sink after each rinse.
4. Block residual binding capacity of wells by filling all wells with PBS-BSA-Tween and incubating for 30 min at room temperature.
5. Rinse the plates 5× over a sink by filling all wells with PBS-Tween from a plastic squirt bottle. Flick the PBS-Tween into the sink after each rinse. After the last wash, remove residual PBS-Tween by laying the plates face down on paper towels for several seconds.

6. Dilute antigen (both standard antigen as a positive control and a tested antigen) in PBS-BSA-Tween (optimal range is from 0.1 to 1000 ng/ml).
7. Add 100 µl of diluted antigen into antibody-coated wells and incubate.
8. Rinse the plates 5× as described in Step 5.
9. Add 100 µl of test samples diluted in PBS-BSA-Tween to each well. Cover the plates and incubate.
10. Rinse the plates 5× as described in Step 5.
11. Add 100 µl of enzyme-conjugated antibody diluted in PBS-BSA-Tween to each well. Cover the plates and incubate.
12. Rinse the plates 5× as described in Step 5.
13. Add 100 µl of substrate solution to each well, cover the plates, and incubate them for 1 hr at room temperature in the dark. Check the visualization occasionally. Read the reaction on ELISA reader using the appropriate filter.
14. Prepare a standard curve from data obtained from antigen standards.
15. Interpolate the concentration of antigen in the test samples from that standard curve.

Comments

1. The optimal concentration of specific antibody and enzyme-conjugated antibody should be determined in a pilot experiment by criss-cross serial dilution analysis.
2. Covered antibody-coated plates can be stored at 4°C for several months. Do not let them dry out.
3. The optimal incubation time in Step 13 depends on the type of enzyme-substrate combination and on the concentration of antibody in tested samples. Stop the reaction (either by reading or by adding stopping reagent) when positive wells reach desired intensity.

III. Direct cellular ELISA[3]

This technique is used for quantitative evaluation of cell-surface determinants using existing enzyme-conjugated antibodies specific for that particular surface marker. Unbound antibody is washed away and a substrate is added for visualization.

Materials and reagents

- ELISA reader
- Enzyme-conjugated antibody
- 96-well U-bottom microtiter plates (Immulon; Dynatech)
- Substrate

- Cells
- PBS containing 0.05% Tween 20 (PBS-Tween)
- Multichannel pipette
- Carbonate-bicarbonate buffer, pH 9.6
- Plastic squirt bottle
- Paper towels
- 15-ml conical centrifuge tubes
- RPMI 1640 medium with 5% FCS
- Vortex

Protocol

1. Prepare cell suspension in RPMI 1640 medium containing 5% FCS and adjust cell density to 2.5×10^5 cells/ml.
2. Dispense 100 µl of the diluted cell suspension into each well. Centrifuge the plate at 450*g* for 2 min at 4°C. Decant the supernatant and gently mix the plate using a vortex to disrupt the pellet.
3. Add 100 µl of the enzyme-antibody conjugate diluted in PBS-Tween into each well and incubate for 2 hr at 4°C.
4. Centrifuge the plate at 450*g* for 2 min at 4°C. Decant the supernatant and gently mix the plate to disrupt the pellet. Resuspend the cells in 200 µl of PBS-Tween. Repeat twice.
5. Add 100 µl of substrate and incubate until the reaction has reached the desired levels at room temperature in the dark.
6. Read the reaction on an ELISA reader using the appropriate filter.

Comments

1. The method is suitable for cell lines or homogenous populations of cells.
2. One can easily convert this method into an indirect ELISA by either substituting unlabeled antibody for the enzyme-conjugated antibody, followed by a second incubation with Ig-specific enzyme-conjugated antibody, or by substituting biotinylated antibody for the enzyme-conjugated antibody, followed by a second incubation with an avidin-enzyme conjugate.
3. The optimal concentration of cells should be determined in a pilot experiment. The most common concentration is in the range of 1 to 5×10^5 cells/ml.
4. The optimal incubation time in Step 5 depends on the type of enzyme-substrate combination and on the concentration of antibody in the test samples. Stop the reaction (either by reading or by adding stopping reagent) when positive wells reach desired intensity.

5. Some types of cells express substantial levels of alkaline phosphatase. A pilot experiment measuring the spontaneous level of alkaline phosphatase (cells and substrate only) must be performed. If these levels are too high, another enzyme-substrate combination must be used.
6. Do not fix the cells unless it is known that the particular surface determinant retains its antigenicity after fixation. In that case, use a 0.5% glutaraldehyde solution in PBS and incubate for 30 min at room temperature.
7. It is also possible to incubate the cells in wells for 24 hr at 37°C (Step 1). In that case, incubate under sterile conditions.

IV. ELISPOT assay[4-7]

The antibodies released from specific antibody-secreting cells are immobilized at the point of release via attachment to an underlying solid phase to which antigens have been chemically conjugated. The captured antibody is subsequently visualized by the application of enzyme-conjugated antibody and an enzyme substrate. Cell products secreted by a single cell generate spots that are permanent. The colored end product is very stable and can be enumerated later. This method is more sensitive than conventional plaque techniques and overcomes their possible disadvantages such as batch-to-batch variations in the susceptibility of target erythrocytes. Recent modifications have improved the sensitivity of the ELISPOT technique such that cells producing as few as 100 molecules of the test protein per second can be detected. The ELISPOT technique can be used for detection of cells secreting antibodies against any antigen, soluble or particulate, that can be absorbed onto a solid surface. This method can be easily modified for enumeration of cytokine-secreting cells[6] by substitution of an anti-Ig antibody with an anti-cytokine antibody.[8]

Materials and reagents

- 24-well tissue culture plates
- Antigen
- Carbonate-bicarbonate buffer, pH 9.6
- Cell suspension
- PBS
- Tween 20 (Sigma)
- PBS containing 1% BSA, 0.05% Tween 20, and 0.02% NaN_3 (PBS-Tween)
- PBS
- Antibodies
- Dulbecco's PBS containing calcium and magnesium, with 1 % BSA
- Substrate
- Agarose (Type 1; Sigma)
- Humidified chamber

Protocol

1. Coat wells with 1 ml of a 2 mg/ml solution of antigen in carbonate-bicarbonate buffer. Incubate overnight at 4°C. Wash 3× with PBS-Tween and 2× with PBS.
2. Add 1 ml cell solution (1 × 10^6cells/ml in Dulbecco's PBS with Ca^{2+}, Mg^{2+} and 1% BSA). Incubate for 2 hr at 37°C in a humidified chamber. Wash 3× with PBS-Tween.
3. Add 1 ml of an appropriate dilution of antibody (use rabbit anti-mouse for mouse cells) in PBS-Tween to each well and incubate for 2 hr at 37°C. Wash 3× with PBS-Tween.
4. Add 1 ml of appropriate dilution of antibody (anti-rabbit in this case; diluted in PBS-Tween) conjugated to an enzyme. Incubate for 2 hr at 37°C. Wash 3× with PBS-Tween.
5. Add 1 ml warm (40°C) agarose-substrate mixture (3% [w/v] stock solution of warm agarose is mixed with substrate solution to a final concentration of 0.6%) to each well. Allow 1 min for it to harden. Incubate for 30 to 60 min at 37°C.
6. Enumerate the macroscopic dots.

V. Two-color ELISPOT[9]

This assay is a modification of the ELISPOT technique in which a combination of two immunoenzymatic reactions, resulting in two different colors, makes it possible to measure two antigenically distinct antibodies secreted from a group of cells.

Materials and reagents

- 96-well nitrocellulose-bottom Millititer HA plates (Millipore)
- PBS
- Paper towels
- Cell suspension
- Two different antibodies (e.g., anti-IgG and anti-IgA) conjugated to two different enzymes
- Appropriate substrates
- PBS
- PBS containing 0.05% Tween 20 (PBS-Tween)
- PBS containing 0.05% Tween 20 and 1% FCS
- 0.05 *M* Tris-buffered saline, pH 8.0
- RPMI 1640 medium with 5% FCS
- CO_2 incubator
- Stereomicroscope

Protocol

1. Dilute antigen in PBS to a concentration of 2 μg/ml and add 100 μl of the solution into each well of a plate. Incubate overnight at 4°C.
2. Wash 3× with PBS.
3. Dry the outer surface of the nitrocellulose membrane with absorbent paper towels.
4. Fill each well with 0.2 ml RPMI 1640 medium with 5% FCS and incubate the plate for 30 min at 37°C.
5. Decant the medium and add 0.1 ml of cell suspension (10^5 cells/well) in RPMI 1640 medium with 5% FCS. Incubate for 4 hr at 37°C in a CO_2 incubator.
6. Wash the plates 3× with PBS and then 3× with PBS-Tween. Incubate the plates in PBS-Tween for 5 min.
7. Decant the PBS-Tween and again dry the outer surface of the nitrocellulose membrane with absorbent paper towels.
8. Add 0.1 ml PBS-Tween with 1% FCS and a mixture of two antibodies (e.g., anti-IgA-alkaline phosphatase and anti-IgG-horseradish peroxidase), respectively, or vice versa, to each well.
9. Incubate for 3 hr at room temperature or overnight at 4°C.
10. Wash the plate 4× with PBS and immerse in 0.05 *M* Tris-buffered saline (pH 8.0), for 5 min prior to development.
11. Decant the buffer and dry again the outer surface of the nitrocellulose membrane with absorbent paper towels.
12. Add 0.1 ml of the first substrate into each well and incubate for 15 min at room temperature. Wash once with PBS and dry again the outer surface of the nitrocellulose membrane with absorbent paper towels.
13. Add 0.1 ml of the second substrate into each well and incubate for an additional 10 min at room temperature. Rinse the plate thoroughly with tap water.
14. Allow the plate to dry and evaluate the individual wells for presence of blue and red spots under low magnification.

Comments

1. Coated plates can be stored for several weeks at 4°C filled with coating solution, or for several months at –20°C after decanting the coating solution. Do not let them dry out.
2. Too long an incubation time in Steps 12 and 13 might result in excessive background staining. Check control wells without cell suspension and adjust the time accordingly.

VI. Labeling of antibodies with alkaline phosphatase[10]

Materials and reagents

- Antibody
- PBS
- Alkaline phosphatase in NaCl solution (Sigma)
- 25% glutaraldehyde, EM grade (Sigma)
- 100 m*M* lysine and 100 m*M* ethanolamine in PBS
- Blocking buffer
- 10-ml Sephadex G-25 column (Pharmacia)
- 0.2-µm filter
- Small plastic tubes
- *p*-Nitrophenyl phosphate substrate (NPP; Sigma)
- $NaCO_3$
- $MgCl_2$
- Fraction collector

Protocol

1. Prepare a 1:3 mixture of antibody and alkaline phosphatase in PBS at greater than 0.2 mg/ml total protein concentration.
2. Add 25% glutaraldehyde to a 0.2% final concentration while vortexing. Incubate for 2 hr at room temperature. Stop reaction by adding an equal volume of blocking buffer.
3. Desalt the antibody by passing through a Sephadex G-25 column in blocking buffer. The Sephadex G-25 volume should be 10 times larger than antibody volume. Collect fractions that are one half the antibody volume.
4. Test individual fractions by adding 2 µl into small tubes containing 0.5 ml NPP substrate (3 m*M* NPP in 0.05 *M* $NaCO_3$ and 0.05 m*M* $MgCl_2$). Pool the first five fractions that strongly hydrolyze NPP.
5. Dilute the pool 1:2 in blocking buffer, filter through a 0.2-µm filter, and store at 4°C for up to 1 year.

VII. Alternate method for labeling of antibodies with alkaline phosphatase[11]

Materials and reagents

- Antibody
- 50% glutaraldehyde, EM grade (Sigma)
- 0.5 *M* Tris, pH 8
- PBS
- Bovine serum albumin (BSA)

- NaN_3
- Dialysis tube
- Alkaline phosphatase in NaCl solution (Sigma)

Protocol

1. Mix 2 mg antibody with 5 mg alkaline phosphatase and place the mixture into a dialysis tube. Dialyze overnight at 4°C against PBS.
2. Remove from the dialysis tube and measure the volume. Add glutaraldehyde to a final concentration of 2% (v/v). Incubate for 2 hr at 4°C with continuous mixing.
3. Transfer the mixture into a dialysis tube and dialyze overnight at 4°C against PBS.
4. Dialyze overnight at 4°C against 0.5 *M* Tris (pH 8).
5. Remove from the dialysis tube and dilute to 4 ml with 0.5 *M* Tris containing 1% BSA and 0.2% NaN_3.
6. Store in the dark at 4°C.

VIII. Labeling of antibodies with horseradish peroxidase[12]

This method may be also used for labeling of antibodies with alkaline phosphatase.

Material and reagents

- Horseradish peroxidase (HRP; Sigma)
- PBS
- 50% glutaraldehyde, EM grade (Sigma)
- Saline
- Antibody
- Carbonate-bicarbonate buffer, pH 9.5
- 0.2 *M* lysine
- Saturated ammonium sulfate (see Chapter 9)
- Human serum albumin (HSA)
- 0.22-μm syringe filter
- Dialysis tube

Protocol

1. Dissolve 10 mg HRP in 0.2 ml PBS containing 1.25% (v/v) glutaraldehyde. Incubate overnight at room temperature with constant mixing.
2. Remove the unreacted glutaraldehyde by dialysis overnight at 4°C against normal saline.
3. Dilute the antibody to a 5 mg/ml concentration with saline.

4. Mix 1 ml activated HRP with 1 ml antibody solution. Add 0.1 ml carbonate-bicarbonate buffer and incubate overnight at 4°C.
5. Add 0.1 ml of 0.2 *M* lysine and mix for 2 hr at room temperature.
6. Dialyze overnight at 4°C against PBS.
7. Precipitate the HRP-conjugated antibody by adding an equal volume of saturated ammonium sulfate. Spin down the precipitate by centrifugation at 2000*g* for 20 min at 4°C and remove the supernatant.
8. Resuspend the precipitate in 1 ml of PBS.
9. Dialyze the conjugate for 48 hr at 4°C against two changes of PBS.
10. Centrifuge the conjugate at 10,000*g* for 30 min at 4°C to remove any sediment.
11. Add HSA up to 1% (w/v) and filter through a 0.22-μm syringe filter.
12. Store at –20°C.

IX. Labeling of antibodies by a periodate method[13]

Materials and reagents

- Antibody
- Alkaline phosphatase (Sigma) or horseradish peroxidase (Sigma)
- 0.3 *M* Na_2CO_3, pH 8.1
- 0.01 *M* Na_2CO_3, pH 9.5
- 1-Fluoro-2,4-dinitrobenzene (Sigma)
- Ethanol
- Bovine serum albumin (BSA)
- 0.08 *M* sodium periodate
- 0.16 *M* ethylene glycol
- PBS
- Sodium borohydride
- Sephadex G200 (Pharmacia)
- Column
- Dialysis tubing
- Fraction collector
- Spectrophotometer

Protocol

1. Dialyze 5 ml alkaline phosphatase or horseradish peroxidase against 0.3 *M* Na_2CO_3 buffer (pH 8.1), overnight at 4°C.
2. Add 0.1 ml of a 1% solution of 1-fluoro-2,4-dinitrobenzene (dissolved in absolute ethanol) to the dialyzed solution and mix gently for 60 min at room temperature.
3. Add 1 ml of 0.08 *M* sodium periodate (freshly prepared) and gently mix for 30 min at room temperature.

4. Add 1 ml of 0.15 *M* ethylene glycol and mix gently for 60 min at room temperature.
5. Dialyze against 0.01 *M* Na_2CO_3 (pH 9.5), overnight at 4°C.
6. Dialyze your antibody against 0.01 *M* Na_2CO_3 (pH 9.5), overnight at 4°C.
7. Mix the dialyzed antibody and 3 ml of the enzyme-aldehyde solution (Step 5) and mix for 3 hr at room temperature.
8. Add 5 mg sodium borohydride and incubate for 3 hr at 4°C.
9. Dialyze the conjugate against PBS for 24 hr at 4°C.
10. Apply the conjugate to the Sephadex G200 column. Elute with PBS at a flow rate of 5 ml/hr. Collect 2-ml fractions and check the absorbance at OD_{280}. The first peak contains the conjugate.
11. Store at –20°C in 1% BSA.

X. Labeling of antibodies with β-D-galactosidase[14]

Materials and reagents

- Purified antibody
- β-D-Galactosidase (Sigma)
- N,N'-*o*-phenylendimaleimide (Aldrich)
- Bovine serum albumn (BSA)
- $MgCl_2$
- 1 *M* NaOH
- 0.01 *M* Sodium phosphate buffer, pH 7.0
- 0.1 *M* Sodium acetate buffer, pH 5.0
- Sephadex G25 column (Pharmacia)
- Sephadex 6B column (Pharmacia)
- Water bath
- Fraction collector
- Spectrophotometer
- Dialysis tubing
- NaCl
- NaN_3

Protocol

1. Dissolve the antibody in 0.1 *M* sodium acetate buffer (pH 5.0), to a concentration of 3 mg/ml.
2. Add 2 ml of the antibody solution dropwise into 1 ml of a saturated solution of N,N'-*o*-phenylendimaleimide in 0.1 *M* sodium acetate buffer (pH 5.0), at 4°C. Incubate at 30°C for 20 min.
3. Equilibrate a Sephadex G25 column with 0.1 *M* sodium acetate buffer (pH 5.0). Apply an antibody solution and collect 1-ml fractions. Check

the antibody concentration at OD_{280} and pool antibody-containing fractions.

4. Adjust the pH of the isolated dimaleimide-treated antibody to 6.5 using a sodium phosphate buffer (pH 7.0).
5. Dialyze β-D-Galactosidase against 0.01 *M* sodium phosphate buffer (pH 7.0), overnight at 4°C. Store in 0.01 *M* sodium phosphate buffer (pH 7.0), supplemented with 0.5% BSA and 1 m*M* $MgCl_2$.
6. Incubate the dimaleimide-treated antibody with β-D-Galactosidase (1:1 w/w ratio) at 30°C for 20 min in 0.1 *M* sodium acetate buffer (pH 5.0).
7. Adjust the pH to 7.0 and apply to a Sepharose 6B column equilibrated with 0.01 *M* sodium phosphate buffer (pH 7.0), containing 0.1 *M* NaCl, 1 m*M* $MgCl_2$, 0.01% BSA, and 0.1% NaN_3.

References

1. Mishell, R.I. and Dutton, R.W., Immunization of normal mouse spleen cells in suspensions *in vitro*, *Science*, 153, 1004, 1966.
2. Engvall, E. and Perlman, P., Enzyme-linked immunosorbent assay (ELISA): Quantitative assay of immunoglobulin G, *Immunochemistry*, 8, 871, 1971.
3. Porstman, B. and Porstman, T., Chromogenic substrates for enzyme immunoassays, in *Nonisotopic Immunoassays*, Ngo, T.T., Ed., Plenum Press, New York, 1988, 57.
4. Feit, C., Bartal, A.H., Tauber, G., Dymbort, G., and Hirshaut, Y., An enzyme-linked immunosorbent assay (ELISA) for the detection of monoclonal antibodies recognizing antigens expressed on viable cells, *J. Immunol. Methods*, 58, 301, 1983.
5. Sedgwick, J.D. and Holt, P.G., A solid-phase immunoenzymatic technique for the enumeration of specific antibody-secreting cells, *J. Immunol. Methods*, 57, 301, 1983.
6. Czerkinsky, C., Nilsson, L.A., Nygren, H., Ouchterlony, O., and Tarkowski, A., A solid-phase enzyme-linked immunospot (ELISPOT) assay for enumeration of specific antibody-secreting cells, *J. Immunol. Methods*, 65, 109, 1983.
7. Czerkinsky, C., Anderson, G., Ferrua, B., Nordstom, I., Quiding, M., Eriksson, K., Larson, L., Hellstrand, K., and Ekre, H., Detection of human cytokine-secreting cells in distinct anatomical compartments, *Immunol. Rev.*, 119, 5, 1991.
8. Czerkinsky, C. and Sedgwick, J., Enzyme-linked immunospot (ELISPOT) assays for detection of specific antibody-secreting cells, in *Methods of Immunological Analysis*, Masseyeff, R.F., Albert, W.H., and Staines, N.A., Eds., VCH Verlagsgesellschaft, Weinheim, 1993, 504.
9. Sedwick, J., Cooke, A., Dorries, R., Hutchings, P., and Schwender, S., Detection and enumeration of single antibody- or cytokine-secreting cells by the ELISA-plaque (ELISPOT) assay, in *Laboratory Methods in Immunology*, Vol. 1., Zola, H., Ed., CRC Press, Boca Raton, FL, 1990, 103.
10. Czerkinsky, C., Moldoveanu, Z., Mestecky, J., Nilsson, L A., and Ouchterlony, O., A novel two colour ELISPOT assay. I. Simultaneous detection of distinct types of antibody-secreting cells, *J. Immunol. Methods*, 115, 31, 1988.

11. Hornbeck, P., Antibody detection and preparation, in *Current Protocols in Immunology,* Coligan, J.E., Kruisbeek, A.M., Margulies, D.H., Shevach, E.M., and Strober, W., Eds., Greene Publishing and Wiley InterScience, New York, 1991, 2.0.1.
12. Avrameas, S., Coupling of enzymes to proteins with glutaraldehyde, *Immunochemistry,* 6, 43, 1969.
13. Avrameas, S. and Ternynck, T., Peroxidase labelled antibody and Fab' conjugates with enhanced intracellular penetration, *Immunochemistry,* 8, 1175, 1971.
14. Nakane, P.K. and Kawaoi, A., Peroxidase-labelled antibody; a new method of conjugation, *J. Histochem. Cytochem.,* 22, 1084, 1974.
15. Kato, K., Fukui, H., Hamaguchi, Y., and Ishikawa, E., Enzyme-linked immunoassay: conjugation of the Fab' fragment of rabbit IgG with β-D-Galactosidase from *E. coli* and its use in immunoassay, *J. Immunol.,* 116, 1554, 1976.

chapter eleven

Buffers and media

Contents

ACK lysing buffer

NH_4Cl	8.29 g
$KHCO_3$	1 g
Na_2EDTA	37.2 mg

Add 800 ml H_20 and adjust pH to 7.2 with 1 *N* HCl. Add H_2O to 1000 ml. Filter through a 0.2-μm filter and store at room temperature.

Hemolytic Gey's solution

Stock A:

NH_4Cl	35 g
KCl	1.85 g
$Na_2HPO_4 \cdot 12\ H_2O$	1.5 g
KH_2PO_4	0.12 g
Glucose	5 g
Phenol red	60 mg
H_2O	1000 ml

Autoclave.

Stock B:

$MgCl_2$	0.42 g
$MgSO_4$	0.14 g
$CaCl_2$	0.34 g
H_2O	1000 ml

Autoclave.

Stock C:

$NaHCO_3$	2.25 g
H_2O	100 ml

Autoclave.

Dispase/DNAase solution

Prepare 60 ml dispase grade II (Boehringer Mannheim) in RPMI 1640 at 1 mg/ml. Add 0.06 ml of a 5 mg/ml DNAase grade II (Boehringer Mannheim). Keep on ice.

1X Gey's solution

20 parts Stock A
5 parts Stock B
5 parts Stock C
70 parts sterile H_2O

Tris-buffered ammonium chloride

Stock A:

NH_4Cl	8.3 g
H_2O	1000 ml

Stock B:
Tris base: dissolve 20.6 g Tris base in 900 ml H_2O; adjust pH to 7.65 with HCl. Add water to 1000 ml.

Working solution:
Mix 90 ml of Stock A with 10 ml Stock B; adjust pH to 7.2

Glucose-phosphate-buffered saline (G-PBS)

Dextrose	10 g
NaCl	8.2 g
1.0 *M* phosphate buffer, pH 7.6	10 ml
H_2O	1000 ml

1.0 M phosphate buffer, pH 7.6

Stock A:

KH_2PO_4	136.1 g
H_2O	1000 ml

Stock B:

$Na_2HPO_4 \cdot 7\ H_2O$	268.1 g/l
(Warm to 45°C to dissolve)	
H_2O	1000 ml

Mix 90 ml of Stock A with 910 ml of Stock B. Adjust to pH 7.6 with Stock B.

0.3 M phosphate buffer

KH_2PO_4	40.7 g	270 ml
$Na_2HPO_4 \cdot 7\ H_2O$	80.4 g	930 ml

Adjust to pH 6.8 and store at 4°C.

Borate-buffered saline (BBS)

Put the following ingredients into a 4-l glass beaker and heat on stirrer hot plate:

NaCl	43.9 g
H_3BO_3	61.9 g
H_2O	5000 ml

Adjust to pH 8.0 with 0.15 *M* NaOH. Add H_2O up to a total volume of 6 liters.

Borate-buffered saline (BBS) (for Biotin label)

Place the following ingredients into a 4-l glass beaker and heat on stirred hot plate (for 6 l):

Na tetraborate $\cdot$ 10 H_2O	57.24 g
NaCl	26.28 g
H_3BO_3	37.1 g

After everything is dissolved, add to 8-l carboy and fill to 6 l with H_2O. Adjust pH to 8.43 and filter before using. Store at room temperature.

Percoll mix solution

10X PBS	45 ml
0.6 *N* HCl	3 ml
H_2O	132 ml

Adjust to pH 7.0 to 7.2.

Türk solution

Acetic acid, concentrated	3 ml
1% crystal violet in H_2O	3 ml
H_2O	294 ml

DMEM medium (DMEM with high glucose)

MOPS [3-(*N*-morpholino)propanesulfonic acid]	2.09 g
2-Mercaptoethanol	0.05 m*M*
L-glutamine	216 mg
L-arginine	116 mg
L-asparagine	36 mg
Folic acid	6 mg

Add H_2O up to a total volume of 1000 ml.

Labeling buffer

Place the following ingredients into a 4-l glass beaker and heat on stirred hot plate. After dissolution, add to 20-l carboy and fill to 10 l with H_2O.

Boric acid	30.9 g
NaCl	116.88 g

Adjust pH to 9.2 and store at 4°C.

Dialyzing buffer

Tris-HCl	157.6 g
NaN_3	10 g
NaCl	116.88 g

Adjust pH to 7.4 and store at 4°C.

Carbonate-bicarbonate buffer

Na_2CO_3	1.59 g
$NaHCO_3$	2.93 g
NaN_3	0.2 g
H_2O	1000 ml

Adjust pH to 9.6. Store at 4°C for no longer than 2 weeks.

5X EGTA buffer

EGTA	7.61 g
KCl	8.95 g
H_2O	1000 ml

Store at 4°C.

Calcium-EGTA buffers

5X EGTA buffer
$CaCO_3$
1 *M* $CaCl_2$, pH 8.0
1 *M* HEPES
1 *M* HCl
120 m*M* KCl

1. Add $CaCO_3$ to 20 ml of 5X EGTA buffer. Add enough $CaCO_3$ to titrate 80% of the EGTA. Heat and stir until dissolved. Adjust to pH 9.2 with 1 *M* HCl. This buffer is 4X calcium/5X EGTA.
2. Slowly add 1 *M* $CaCl_2$ to 4 ml of 4X calcium/5X EGTA with constant measuring of the pH levels at room temperature. Stop adding $CaCl_2$ when pH stops decreasing. Calculate the number of millimoles of $CaCl_2$ required and add the appropriate amount of 1 *M* $CaCl_2$ to 10 ml of 4X calcium/5X EGTA. This buffer is 5X calcium/EGTA buffer.
3. Add 1 *M* HEPES to 20 m*M* final and 1 *M* $MgCl_2$ to 1 m*M* final to the 5X calcium/EGTA buffer. Adjust to the desired pH with 1 *M* HCl and bring to 50 ml with 120 m*M* KCl. This buffer is 1X calcium/EGTA ($K_2CaEGTA$) buffer.
4. Add 1 *M* HEPES to 20 m*M* final and 1 m*M* $MgCl_2$ to 1 m*M* final to 10 ml of 5X EGTA buffer. Adjust to the same pH as previous buffer and add 120 m*M* KCl up to 50 ml. This buffer is 1X EGTA (K_2H_2EGTA) buffer.
5. To obtain a buffer of a desired Ca^{2+} concentration, determine the required amounts of total calcium and EGTA and mix the 1X EGTA and calcium/EGTA buffers in the appropriate ratio.

Hanks' balanced salt solution with calcium and magnesium

$CaCl_2$	0.11 g
$MgCl_2$	95.21 mg
FCS	10 ml
H_2O	1000 ml

Store at 4°C.

Veronal buffered saline

NaCl	8.77 g
$MgCl_2$	76.17 mg
$CaCl_2$	33.3 mg
Sodium barbital	8.24 mg

NaN_3	0.2 g
H_2O	1000 ml

Adjust pH to 7.4 and store at 4°C.

Blocking buffer

Borate buffered saline containing:

EDTA	0.292 g
Tween 20	0.5 ml
BSA	2.5 g
NaN_3	0.5 g
$MgCl_2$	0.238 g
H_2O	1000 ml

Cacodylate buffer

Cacodylic acid	38.6 g

Add 900 ml H_2O and adjust pH to 6.9 with 10 *M* NaOH. Bring volume to 1000 ml and store at 4°C. **Cacodylic acid is highly poisonous.**

Staining solution

0.5% Coomassie Brilliant Blue R-250
40% Ethanol
10% Glacial acetic acid
50% H_2O

Store at room temperature.

Destaining solution

15% Ethanol
5% Glacial acetic acid
80% H_2O

Store at room temperature.

0.1 M Sodium acetate buffer

Stock A:

Sodium acetate	51.7 g
H_2O	750 ml

Stock B:

Glacial acetic acid	21.7 ml
H_2O	728.3 ml

Stock C:

3 *M* NaCl	1,000 ml

Lower the pH of Stock A with Stock B to pH 4.1. Mix 200 ml Stock A with 30 ml Stock C and 770 ml H_2O. Readjust the pH with Stock B to pH 4.1

Acetate/EDTA buffer

3 m*M* EDTA-HCl	0.9 g
0.1 *M* sodium acetate	13.6 g
H_2O	1000 ml

Adjust to pH 5.5 with glacial acetic acid.

Borate buffers: pH 8.5, 9.0, and 10.0

0.1 M, pH 8.5:

Boric acid	18.55 g
H_2O	3000 ml

0.16 M, pH 9.0:

Sodium borate ($Na_2B_4O_7$)	6.1 g
NaCl	0.76 g
H_2O	100 ml

0.1 M, pH 10.0:

Boric acid	0.618 g
H_2O	100 ml

0.1 M Diethanolamine buffer, pH 9.8

0.2 *M* Diethanolamine	50 ml
0.2 *M* HCl	5.74 ml
H_2O	44.26 ml

DTNB solution

Dissolve 39.6 mg DTNB in 10 ml of 0.05 *M* phosphate buffer, pH 8.0. Adjust to pH 8.0 with 0.1 *M* NaOH if necessary. Prepare fresh for each assay.

0.3% Glutaraldehyde

25% Glutaraldehyde	1.2 ml
Borate buffer, pH 10.0	98.8 ml

Prepare immediately before use.

0.01 M Phosphate buffer, pH 7.0

KH_2PO_4	1.36 g
H_2O	to 1000 ml

Adjust pH with 10 M NaOH.

0.05 M Phosphate buffer: pH 6.0 and 8.0

KH_2PO_4	6.8 g
H_2O	to 1000 ml

Adjust pH with 10 *M* NaOH.

0.05 M Tris-buffered saline

0.05 *M* Tris-HCl	0.8 g
1.5 *M* NaCl	9 g
H_2O	100 ml

Adjust to pH 8.0 and store at room temperature.

Dulbecco's PBS with Ca^{2+}, Mg^{2+}, and BSA

Dulbecco's PBS	990 ml
$CaCl_2$	0.11 g
$MgCl_2$	95.21 mg
BSA	10 ml

Balanced salt solution (BSS)

The 10X BSS is made up as two stock solutions.

Stock 1:

Dextrose	10 g
KH_2PO_4	0.6 g
$Na_2HPO_4 \cdot 7\ H_2O$	3.58 g
0.5% Phenol red solution	20 ml

Dissolve and bring to 1000 ml with distilled water.

Stock 2:

$CaCl_2 \cdot 2\ H_2O$	1.86 g
KCl	4 g
NaCl	80 g
$MgCl_2$, anhydrous	1.04 g
$MgSO_4 \cdot 7\ H_2O$	2 g

1. Dissolve and bring to 1000 ml with distilled water.
2. Test the 10X stocks by making a sample of 1X BSS. Mix 10 ml of Stock 1 and 10 ml Stock 2 and bring to 100 ml with distilled water. The 1X BSS should be at pH 7.2 to 7.4 and have a conductivity of 14 to 16 mS.
3. 2X and 1X BSS are obtained by appropriate dilutions of the 10X stocks with distilled water. The 2X and 1X BSS can be sterilized by passage through a 0.22-μm filter.

Comments

1. Store the 10X stock at 4°C.
2. Make nonsterile 1X BSS for the hemolytic assays just prior to use. Discard the remaining 1X BSS after use.
3. Prepare sterile 2X and 1X BSS immediately after preparing the 10X stocks. Then incubate the filtered BSS at 37°C for 1 week prior to use to detect bacterial contamination. The sterile BSS is stored at room temperature and appears to have an indefinite shelf-life.

Texas red labeling buffer

$NaHCO_3$	16.80 g
NaCl	8.76 g
H_2O	to 1000 ml

Dissolve and adjust pH to 9.0 with 1N NaOH. Store at 4°C.

chapter twelve

Commercial sources

Accurate Chemical and Scientific
300 Shames Drive
Westbury, NY 11590
Tel: (800) 645-6264
Fax: (516) 997-4948
www.accurate-assi-leeches.com

Advanced Magnetics, Inc.
61 Mooney Street
Cambridge, MA 02138-1038
Tel: (800) 343-1346
Fax: (617) 497-6927
www.advancedmagnetics.com

Aldrich Chemical Co., Inc.
940 W. St. Paul Avenue
Milwaukee, WI 53233
Tel: (800) 558-9160
(414) 273-3850
Fax: (800) 962-9591
(414) 273-4979
www.sigma-aldrich.com

Amac, Inc.
160B Larrabee Road
Westbrook, ME 04092
Tel: (800) 458-5060
Fax: (207) 854-0116

Amersham Pharmacia Biotech
800 Centennial Avenue
P.O. Box 1327
Piscataway, NJ 08855-1327
Tel: (800) 526-3593
Fax: (877) 295-8102
www.apbiotech.com

Amgen Biologicals
Amgen Inc. (Headquarters)
Amgen Center
Thousand Oaks, CA 91320-1799
Tel: (805) 447-1000
Fax: (805) 447-1010
www.amgen.com

Amicon Corporation (bought by Millipore)
Scientific Systems Division
21 Hartwell Avenue
Lexington, MA 02173
Tel: (617) 862-7050
www.millipore.com

ATCC (American Type Culture Collection)
10801 University Boulevard
Manassas, VA 20110-2209
Tel: (703) 365-2700
www.atcc.org

BD Biosciences
2350 Qume Drive
San Jose, CA 95131-1807
Tel: (800) 235-5953
Fax: (408) 954-2347
www.bdbiosciences.com

BD Pharmingen and BD Transduction Laboratories
10975 Torreyana Road
San Diego, CA 92121-1106
Tel: (800) 848-6227
(800) 825-5832 Technical Service
FAX: (800) 325-9637
www.bdbiosciences.com

Beckman Coulter, Inc.
4300 N. Harbor Boulevard
P.O. Box 3100
Fullerton, CA 92834-3100
Tel: (714) 871-4848
Fax: (714) 773-8283
www.beckmancoulter.com

Bio-Rad Laboratories
2200 Wright Avenue
Richmond, CA 94804
Tel: (415) 234-4130
www.bio-rad.com

Biosource International
542 Flynn Road
Camarillo, CA 93012
Tel: (805) 987-0086
(800) 242-0607 Technical Service
Fax: (805) 987-3385
www.biosource.com/

Biotech, C-C Biotech Corporation
16766 Espola Road
Poway, CA 92064
Tel: (619) 451-9949
Fax: (619) 487-8138

Biotex Laboratories Inc.
#100, 8905-51 Avenue
Edmonton, Alberta, Canada T6E 5J3
Tel: (800) 661-1426
(403) 448-0621
Fax: (403) 448-0624

BioWhittaker, Inc.
8830 Biggs Ford Road
Walkersville, MD 21793
Tel: (800) 638-8174
(301) 898-7025
Fax: (301) 845-8338
www.biowhittaker.com

Boehringer-Mannheim (*see* Roche Molecular Biochemicals)
www.biochem.boehringer-mannheim.com

Calbiochem-Novabiochem Corporation
P.O. Box 12087
La Jolla, CA 92039-2087
Tel: (800) 854-3417
(619) 450-9600
Fax: (800) 776-0999
www.calbiochem.com

Cedarlane Accurate Chemicals & Scientific Corp.
300 Shames Drive
Westbury, NY 11590
Tel: (800) 645-6264
Fax: (516) 997-4948

Cleveland Scientific
P.O. Box 300
Bath, OH 44210
Tel: (216) 666-7676
Fax: (216) 666-2240

Corning Science Product Division (*see also* Costar)
45 Nagog Park
Acton, MA 01720
Tel: (800) 492-7711
Fax: (978) 492-1112
www.corningcostar.com

Costar
Corporate Headquarters
One Alewife Center
Cambridge, MA 02140
Tel: (800) 492-1110
(617) 868-6200
Fax: (617) 868-2076

Coulter Cytometry (*see* Beckman Coulter, Inc.)
www.coulter.com/

CytRx Corporation
154 Technology Parkway
Technology Park/Atlanta
Norcross, GA 30092
Tel: (770) 368-9500
Fax: (770) 447-8875
www.titermax.com

Dako Corporation
6392 Via Real
Carpinteria, CA 93013
Tel: (800) 235-5743
(805) 566-6655
Fax: (805) 566-6688
www.dakousa.com

Difco Laboratories, Inc.
P.O. Box 1058A
Detroit, MI 48640
Tel: (313) 961-0800
Fax: (313) 462-8517
www.difco.com

Dynal Inc.
5 Delaware Drive
Lake Success, NY 11042
Tel: (800) 638-9416
Fax: (516) 326-3298
www.dynal.net

Dynatech Laboratories, Inc.
900 Slaters Lane
Alexandria, Virginia 22314
Tel: (800) 336-4543
(703) 548-3889

Eastman Fine Chemicals, Eastman Kodak Company
1001 Lee Road, Building 701
Rochester, NY 14650
Tel: (800) 225-5352
(716) 588-2572
Fax: (800) 879-4979
(716) 722-6054

Endogen, Inc. (*see also* Pierce Endogen)
68 Fargo Street
Boston, MA 02210-2122
Tel: (800) 487-4885
(617) 439-3250
Fax: (617) 439-0355
www.endogen.com/

Fisher Scientific
711 Forbes Avenue
Pittsburg, PA 15219
Tel: (800) 766-7000
Fax: (800) 926-1166
www.fishersci.com

FMC Bioproducts
191 Thomaston Street
Rockland, ME 04841
Tel: (800) 341-1574
Fax: (800) 362-5552
www.bioproducts.com

Falcon Products, Becton Dickinson Labware
1950 Williams Drive
Oxnard, CA 93030
Tel: (800) 235-5953
(805) 485-8711

Gibco BRL
Corporate Headquarters
Life Technologies, Inc.
P.O. Box 9418
Gaithersburg, MD 20898
Tel: (800) 828-6686
Fax: (800) 331-2286
www.lifetech.com

Harlan Bioproducts for Science
P.O. Box 29176
Indianapolis, IN 46229
Tel: (800) 9-SCIENCE
(317) 894-7536
Fax: (317) 357-9000
www.harlan.com

HyClone Laboratories
1725 S. State Highway 89-91
Logan, UT 84321
Tel: (800) 492-5663
Fax: (801) 753-4589
www.hyclone.com

ICN Biomedicals, Inc.
3300 Hyland Avenue
Costa Mesa, CA 92626
Tel: (800) 854-0530
Fax: (800) 334-6999
www.icnbiomed.com

Immunotech Corporation (*see* Beckman Coulter, Inc.)

Integra Biosciences
10097 Tyler Place, Suite 10
Ijamsville, MD 21754
Tel: (800) 886-8675
Fax: (301) 874-5799
www.integra-biosciences.com

Intergen Company
Two Manhattanville Road
Purchase, NY 10577
Tel: (800) 431-4505
(914) 694-1700
Fax: (914) 694-1429

Irvine Scientific
2511 Daimler Street
Santa Ana, CA 92705
Tel: (800) 437-5706
Fax: (714) 261-6522
www.irvinesci.com/

Jackson Immunoresearch Laboratories, Inc.
827 West Baltimore Pike
P.O. Box 9
West Grove, PA 19390-0014
Tel: (800) 367-5296
Fax: (215) 869-0171
www.jacksonimmuno.com

The Jackson Laboratory
60 Main Street
Bar Harbor, ME 04609
Tel: (800) 422-6423
Fax: (207) 288-3398
www.jax.org

Millipore Products Division
80 Ashby Road
Bedford, MA 01730
Tel: (800) 645-5476
(781) 533-8622
Fax: (781) 533-8630
www.millipore.com

Miltenyi Biotec, Inc.
1250 Oakmead Park, Suite 210
Sunnyvale, CA 94088
Tel: (800) 367-6227
Fax: (916) 888-8925
www.myltenyibiotec.com

Molecular Probes, Inc.
P.O. Box 22010
Eugene, OR 97402-0414
Tel: (503) 465-8300
Fax: (503) 344-6504
www.probes.com

NEN Life Sciences Products (Perkin Elmer Life Sciences, Inc.)
549 Albany Street
Boston, MA 02118
Tel: (800) 551-2121
www.nen.com

Neuro Probe
16008 Industrial Drive
Gaithersburg, MD 20877
Tel: (301) 417-0014
Fax: (301) 977-5711
www.neuroprobe.com

Nordic Immunological Labs
Drawer 2517
Capistrano Beach, CA 92624
Tel: (800) 554-6655
(714) 498-4467
Fax: (714) 361-0138

Norton Performance Plastic
P.O. Box 3660
Akron, OH 44309

Nunc
200 N. Aurora Road
Naperville, IL 60563
Tel: (800) 288-6862
Fax: (708) 416-2556
www.nunc.nalgenunc.com

Oncogene Science Inc.
106 Charles Lindbergh Boulevard
Uniondale, NY 11553-3649
Tel: (800) 662-2616
Fax: (516) 222-0114
www.oncogene.com

Pacific Bio-Marine Laboratory, Inc.
P.O. Box 1348
Venice, CA 90294
Tel: (310) 822-5757
Fax: (310) 215-1938

PeproTech, Inc.
Princeton Business Park
5 Crescent Avenue, G2
P.O. Box 275
Rocky Hill, NJ 08553
Tel: (800) 436-9910
Fax: (609) 497-0321
www.peprotech.com

Pharmacia LKB Biotechnology (*see* Amersham Pharmacia Biotech)
www.pharmacia.se/ns4index.html

Pharmingen (*see* BD Pharmingen)
www.pharmingen.com

Pierce Endogen
P.O. Box 117
Rockford, IL 61103
Tel: (800) 874-3723
Fax: (800) 842-5007
www.piercenet.com

Polysciences, Inc.
400 Valley Road
Warrington, PA 18976-2590
Tel: (800) 523-2575
(215) 343-6484
Fax: (215) 343-0214
www.polysciences.com

Promega Corporation
2800 Woods Hollow Road
Madison, WI 53711-5399
Tel: (800) 356-9526
(608) 274-4330
Fax: (608) 277-2516
www.promega.com

R & D Systems
614 McKinley Place NE
Minneapolis, MN 55413
Tel: (800) 343-7475
Fax: (612) 379-6580
www.rndsystems.com

Research Products International Corp.
410 N. Business Center Drive
Mount Prospect, IL 60056-2190
Tel: (708) 635-7330
Fax: (708) 635-1177
www.rpicorp.com

Ribi Immunochem Research, Inc. (bought by Corixa)
553 Old Corvallis Road
Hamilton, MT 59840
Tel: (800) 548-7424
(406) 363-6214
Fax: (406) 363-6129
www.corixa.com
www.ribi.com

Roche Molecular Biochemicals
P.O. Box 50414
Indianapolis, IN 46250-0414
Tel: (800) 428-5433
(800) 262-4911 Technical Service
Fax: (800) 428-2883
www.roche.com

Sandoz Pharmaceutical Co.
59 Route 10
East Hanover, NJ 07936
Tel: (800) 526-0175
Fax: (201) 503-6356
www.novartis.com/home
www.sandoz.com

Sarstedt
P.O. Box 468
Newton, NC 28658
Tel: (800) 257-5101
Fax: (704) 465-4003
www.sarstedt.com

Serotec Inc. (USA)
NCSU Centennial Campus
Partners 1, 1017 Main Campus Drive, Suite 2450
Raleigh, NC 27606
Tel: (800) 265-7376
(919) 515-9977
Fax: (919) 515-9980
www.serotec.co.uk

Sigma Chemical Company
P.O. Box 14508
St. Louis, MO 63178
Tel: (800) 325-3010
(314) 771-5750
Fax: (800) 325-5052
(314) 771-5757
www.sigma-aldrich.com

Skatron Instruments, Inc.
108 Terminal Drive
P.O. Box 530
Sterling, VA 20167
Tel: (703) 478-5190
Fax: (703) 478-5197
www.skatron.com

Southern Biotechnology Associates
P.O. Box 26221
Birmingham, AL 35226
Tel: (800) 722-2255
Fax: (205) 945-8765
www.sobio.com

Spectrum Chemical Mfg. Corp.
755 Jersey Avenue
New Brunswick, NJ 08901-3605
Tel: (800) 772-8786
(908) 214-1300
Fax: (800) 525-2299
(908) 220-6553

Spectrum Laboratories, Inc.
18617 Broadwick Street
Rancho Dominguez, CA 90220
Tel: (800) 634-3300
Fax: (800) 445-7330
www.spectrapor.com

Stem Cell Technologies
777 West Broadway, Suite 808
Vancouver, BC, Canada, V5Z 4J7
Tel: (800) 667-0322
(604) 877-0713
Fax: (800) 567-2899
(604) 877-0704
www.stemcell.com

Thomas Scientific
99 High Hill Road at I-295
P.O. Box 99
Swedesboro, NJ 08085-0099
Tel: (800) 345-2100
(609) 467-2000
Fax: (609) 467-3087
www.thomassci.com

Winthrop Pharmaceuticals
Division of Sterling Drug, Inc.
90 Park Avenue
New York, NY 10016
Tel: (212) 907-2000
Fax: (212) 551-7856

Index

E

F

G

H

I

J

K

L

M

N

P

R

S

T

W

For Product Safety Concerns and Information please contact our EU representative GPSR@taylorandfrancis.com Taylor & Francis Verlag GmbH, Kaufingerstraße 24, 80331 München, Germany